Fix Your Posture

Over 70 Effective Exercises to Fix Posture & Stop Back Pain

Fix Your Posture

Over 70 Effective Exercises to Fix Posture & Stop Back Pain

ISBN: 978-1-911267-69-0

Published by **www.fundamental-changes.com**

www.fundamental-changes.com

Facebook: 5sfitnessuk

Instagram: 5s_fitness

Cover Image Copyright: Shutterstock: Africa Studio

Contents

Chapter 1: Introduction   4

Get the Video   7

Chapter 2: Posture   8

Chapter 3: Neck, Upper Back & Shoulder Mobility   12
   Introduction   12
   Neck Stretches   13
   Chest Release Techniques & Stretches   19
   Latissimus Dorsi Release Techniques & Stretches   24
   Thoracic Release Techniques   30
   Thoracic Rotations   33

Chapter 4: Shoulder External Rotation & Retraction Strength   36
   Introduction   36
   Head Retractions & Scapula Pinches   37
   Shoulder External Rotation   40
   Serratus Wall Slides   43
   Band Pull Apart   45
   Band Face Pulls   48
   Band Horizontal Pulls   49
   Bent Over Rows   50
   Single Arm Rows   52
   Bent Over Lateral Raises   54
   Shrugs   55

Chapter 5: Hip & Core Mobility   57
   Introduction   57
   Hip Flexor/Quadriceps Release Techniques & Stretches   57
   Glute/Piriformis Release Techniques & Stretches   61
   Low Back Release Techniques & Stretches   65
   Rectus Abdominis & Oblique Stretches   67
   Hamstring Release Techniques & Stretches   70
   Adductor Release Technique & Stretches   76

Chapter 6: Hip & Core Strength & Stability   81
   Banded Glute Bridges, Frog Pumps & Lateral Band Walks   82
   Banded Psoas March   86
   Dead Bug   87
   Birddog   88
   McGill Curl Up   89
   Ab Roll-Outs   90
   RKC Plank   91
   Side Planks   93
   Pallof Iso Holds   93
   Hip Hinges   95
   Squats   97
   Lunges   100

Chapter 7: Programming   103

Chapter 1: Introduction

When you calculate how many hours a day you spend sitting, it can be quite a shock.

Some people spend an hour or two driving to work each day, the best part of eight hours sitting at their desk, drive home and then spend the rest of the evening on the sofa, equating to twelve or more hours of sitting each day.

Most of us tend to sit a lot and you are probably aware that this isn't great for your body. Yet let's be realistic, how much is it likely to change? Are you going to quit your desk job or stop watching TV in the evening after a hard day's work?

The answer is probably no. We need to find a realistic way to incorporate movement and exercises that help to rectify the problems that prolonged sitting can cause into our routines.

So, what are the problems?

Firstly, excessive sitting means a lack of overall activity levels. This links sitting to obesity, diabetes, and other metabolic diseases associated with weight gain. Worldwide, inactivity causes about 9% of premature deaths. That's over 5 million people dying every year.

Aside from the major, often life-threatening issues, prolonged sitting causes postural problems which have a long list of symptoms such as headaches, and back and neck pain. These postural issues are often referred to as 'desk posture'.

One of the biggest issues with being desk bound is that prolonged sitting tends to promote the activation of the 'tonic' muscles which have the tendency to become tight, and the underuse of the 'phasic' muscles which have the tendency to be longer and less activated. For example, your hip flexors (muscles at the front of your hips) become tight, while your glutes (buttocks) become under-activated.

In this book, I take a thorough approach to developing better posture. Rather than giving you a simplistic 'cure all', I will explain how areas can become problematic, from your hips to your head, and how you can best rectify each issue.

Remember, just because you have neck pain, it doesn't necessarily mean the problem originates in your neck. The body is a kinetic chain, with muscles working together to facilitate movement and support the surrounding structures. If one aspect is off kilter, it can have dramatic effects on the rest.

This may give the impression that you will need an in-depth knowledge of human anatomy and physiology to use this book. I can assure you that rectifying desk posture is actually quite simple. I will give you the best information and exercises for the job. Rectifying and maintaining good posture for the long term, rather than giving you a few quick fixes that won't tackle the root of the problem.

One thing I strongly recommend is to move as much as you can. Your body is made up of 206 bones, 360 joints, and over 600 muscles. Your skin is elastic and your circulatory system and nerves benefit from movement. In short, you are designed to move, so move as much as you can.

Chair & Desk Setup

While the key to keeping your body in good health is movement, sometimes it just isn't feasible to maintain the optimal amount of physical activity. It's therefore important that you have your desk and chair set up in a way that at least tries to minimise the negative effects of desk posture.

Sitting posture will be discussed in greater detail in the next chapter, so here I will just give you a few quick pointers on how to set up your chair and desk.

1. Use a standing desk if you can, with your eyes in line with the top of your monitor.

2. Choose a chair that swivels, has an adjustable seat height, and good lumbar (lower spine) support.

3. If your chair does not properly support your lumbar spine, use a lumbar spine support cushion.

4. Set your chair and monitor height so that with your feet flat to the floor or on a foot rest, your hips are bent at no more than 90 degrees and your eyes are in line with the top of the monitor.

5. Your keyboard and mouse should be at elbow height. Your elbows should be kept into your sides, and bent at around 90 degrees.

6. Use a headset instead of holding a phone to your ear for prolonged periods.

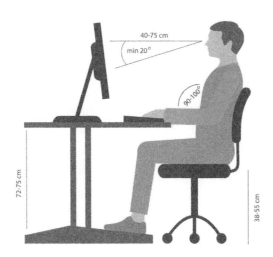

Recommended Equipment

A resistance band and a foam roller are essential to correct your posture and use this book effectively. With just one low-medium tension resistance band and a foam roller, you will be able to carry out most of the exercises to significant effect.

All the equipment listed here can be easily purchased from Amazon.

Resistance Bands (long): I recommend purchasing a yellow, red, and, if you have greater strength, a black band. However, you can effectively work with just one.

- Yellow – Low tension.

- Red – Medium tension (most used band).

- Black – Medium tension, greater than the red band.

Foam Roller: A simple 90cm foam roller is ideal, (30-45cm rollers are also fine). However, if you choose to spend more you can purchase a 'rumble roller' which allows you to get deeper into specific areas.

Massage Ball: You can purchase balls designed specifically for massage, or use a lacrosse ball. Golf balls can be used, but they're often too small to be truly effective. Peanut-shaped massage balls allow you to work both sides of your back, while avoiding pressure on your spine.

Resistance Loop Bands (small band): Small bands are a great tool for hip and shoulder strengthening drills.

Barbell/Dumbbells/Kettlebells: Barbells, dumbbells, and kettlebells are used in a few of the exercises in this book. These pieces of equipment are more likely to be available in a gym. If you have dumbbells, kettlebells or even a barbell at home or in your office, that's great.

Ab Roller: Used for just one core exercise in the book. I highly recommend this piece of equipment as abdominal roll-outs are a truly awesome exercise for your core muscles.

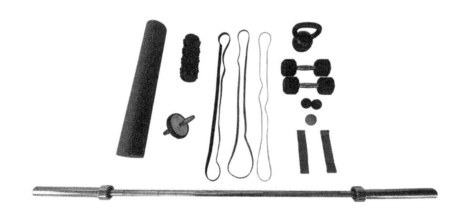

Useful Definitions

Before getting stuck into the exercises, here is a brief overview of some of the terms used in this book.

Range of Motion (ROM): The full movement potential of a joint.

Flexibility: This refers to the range of motion a muscle can achieve passively, essentially the length it can achieve.

Mobility: This refers to how freely a joint can move throughout its full range of motion actively. Flexibility is one (very important) aspect of mobility.

Muscle Tightness: This refers to the muscle-length. If a muscle is tight, then it is shortened. Some muscles have the tendency to be shorter and tighter, while others have the tendency to be longer and less activated.

Muscle Tension: Tension is often considered to be the same as tightness. However, not only tight or overworked muscles become tense. Muscles that are lengthened or weak can also become tense – examples of these will pop up throughout the book.

Reps and sets: "Reps" (repetitions) define the number of times you complete an exercise, and "sets" refers to how many times you will repeat that exercise for the specified number of reps. For example, 5 sets of 3 reps (5x3 – sets first), with 2 minutes rest between sets.

Get the Video

The videos to accompany each exercise are available to download for free from geni.us/fixposture. Simply enrol in the course and you'll have free access to all 34 videos.

geni.us/fixposture

If you type above link into a browser, please notice that there is no "www."

Chapter 2: Posture

In this chapter, I will describe good posture while seated, while standing, and while lying down.

Sitting can exacerbate various postural issues, so if your posture is poor prior to sitting, then you are pretty much setting yourself up for bigger problems.

It's also amazing how many issues poor sleeping positions can cause. When a client comes to me complaining of severe neck pain, they have often slept in an unusual position.

Good posture should align your body so that minimal stress is placed on joints and the supporting muscles, tendons, and ligaments. This results in the stresses of daily life being distributed evenly.

Good posture also allows you to facilitate movement as efficiently as possible, which decreases the stress on your joints, increases your overall performance, and allows for optimal function of your internal organs and nervous system.

Maintaining optimal positioning at all times is, unfortunately, simply not possible. Your body is designed to bend, extend, and rotate, to move into different positions for different tasks. The problem comes when you spend so much time in a single position, that you no longer return to optimal posture once the task is complete.

We have all experienced the negative effects of staying in a static position for too long. To stay pain free, you should maintain a dynamic posture where regular movement occurs.

Movement is vital for your health. However, repeated bending and twisting of your spine, even when unloaded, is not ideal and can lead to issues such as chronic back pain. Movement should predominantly stem from your limbs. Your shoulders and hips are ball-and-socket joints that are designed for a wide variety of movement. In this book, I will not only be teaching you proper positioning, but also proper movement.

Below, I set out my guidelines for good posture. Posture is affected by body type and shape, and these guidelines will help you find what is right for you. Ideally, it will be a position within an optimal range that accommodates your own lifestyle and anatomical structure.

When an individual favours certain muscle groups to achieve an action, it may result in some slight postural deviations. For example, if your job involves repetitive actions, or requires you to be in the same position for prolonged periods, your body will adapt to better facilitate this.

Standing Posture

The standing position is the position in which posture is usually assessed. If I tell an individual I am going to assess their posture, they will quickly pull their head up, their shoulders back, and their stomach in, resulting in an unrealistic assessment. To counter this, I have clients jog on the spot, prior to me abruptly telling them to 'stop'. From there I can see the position that their body naturally falls into.

While standing, the optimal position is to have your feet roughly hip-shoulder width apart, with your knees and hips centred over the middle of your feet halfway between your toes and heels (midfoot).

Your knees should be slightly bent, (often referred to as having 'soft knees'). This allows the musculature of your legs to help support the surrounding structures while reducing stress on your knees and lower back. Maintaining a soft knee position also allows for better circulation through the legs.

Your torso should be balanced over your hips, not leaning forward or back. Your shoulders should be held back and down, with your chest pushed out and your chin held up and back. This allows your ears to sit directly over the centre of your shoulders, which should in turn align vertically with your hips, knees, and midfoot.

Your arms should be held in a controlled manner at your side, once again allowing the musculature to support the surrounding structures.

A great cue for maintaining good posture while standing or walking, is to imagine you are trying to look over a fence that is an inch too high, without going up onto your toes. This will naturally cause you to push your chest out, while retracting your chin and pulling your shoulders back.

TYPES OF STANDING POSTURE

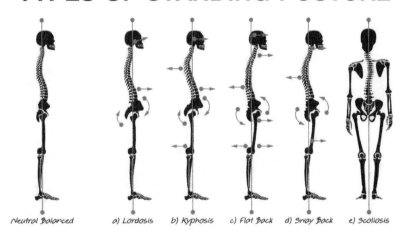

Neutral Balanced   a) Lordosis   b) Kyphosis   c) Flat Back   d) Sway Back   e) Scoliosis

Sitting Posture

When sitting without any back support, your torso should be positioned over your hips.

Your shoulders should be pulled back and down, and your chin should be up and back. This results in your ears falling in line with the centre of your shoulders and hips, just like in a standing position.

The height of your seat should allow your upper legs to rest parallel to the ground, or slope towards the floor. You don't want your knees higher than your hips. This restricts the circulation through your legs and holds your hip flexor muscles in a shortened position, potentially leading to postural issues and lower back pain.

Regular movement is the key to soft tissue health, so your foot position should be comfortable, but changed regularly.

If you are leaning forward slightly it's fine to tuck your feet under the chair, but if you are leaning back on a chair rest, then your feet should be flat on the floor in front of you. If your feet dangle off the chair it will pull your pelvis into an anterior tilt (forward tilt) and result in your core musculature having to compensate.

Spreading your feet out to the front on your heels, will encourage you to slouch. Crossing your legs should also be avoided as it will result in one hip sitting higher than the other. This limits circulation and places extra strain on your spine.

When sitting on a chair with a back rest, the same postural cues should be taken. However, it's important to ensure that you push your bum to the rear of the chair prior to sitting up, which prevents you from slouching.

Remember, prolonged sitting, regardless of how well you are positioned, can potentially cause issues.

Lying Posture

When lying or sleeping, it all comes down to what is comfortable for you. Yes, there are certain sleeping positions which are advised against, such as sleeping on your stomach, as they generally result in poor alignment of your spine and can potentially restrict breathing.

However, if that's the position you've slept in since childhood with no problems, then the likelihood of it changing is slim.

Pillows can be used to help achieve a more supported sleeping position:

- Use a pillow that keeps the cervical spine (neck) in a neutral position

- Back lying - Placing a pillow under your knees will take the stress off your knee joints and your lower back.

- Side lying - Placing a pillow between your legs can help to keep your spine in good alignment.

- Side lying - Hugging a pillow to the front can help to maintain a comfortable position for your shoulders.

- Side lying - A pillow placed behind you can be used to lean back on, which will help to take pressure off your shoulders.

- Stomach sleeping – A long pillow can be used to raise one arm and one leg. This puts you into a more diagonal sleeping position, helping to keep your spine in good alignment.

In the morning, remember that your intervertebral discs (the fluid filled sacks that act as shock absorbers between each vertebra) are at the greatest risk of injury when you first get up.

When you are lying down, gravity does not compress your spine as it does when you are standing, so the amount of fluid within the discs increases. This in turn increases the pressure placed through them when you flex your spine.

To avoid damaging these discs, you should use a controlled roll to one side to get out of bed, rather than the more aggressive 'sit up' action that is commonly used, especially when late for work!

This increase of disc size is the reason why you are slightly taller in the morning, and why it is highly recommended that you mobilise your spine, especially if you are undertaking any resistance training in the morning. The 'cat camel' exercise described later is ideal for this.

Correct Sleep Posture

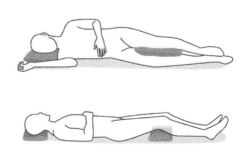

Chapter 3: Neck, Upper Back & Shoulder Mobility

Introduction

In this chapter, I will give you various drills that will release and stretch the upper body muscles that pull you into poor posture. When I use the word release, I am referring to self-myofascial release.

Fascia are the sheets of connective tissue beneath the skin that attach, stabilise, enclose, and separate muscles and other internal organs. It's been proven that muscle fascia plays a major role in muscle tension.

The self-myofascial release techniques I will show you in this book are a method of hands-on therapy that you can perform yourself, usually with a foam roller or massage ball. The aim of these techniques is to use pressure to stimulate a sensory receptor called the Golgi tendon organ that tells the muscle fibers to relax.

These techniques will not stimulate a long-term change in muscle tension by themselves. Instead they will cause a short-term release of muscle tension, which in turn will allow you to gain a more effective stretch to the tissues.

Release techniques and stretching will provide you with short-term relief from excessive tension that might be causing pain or discomfort. The long-term aim is to incorporate these techniques with exercises to strengthen specific muscles and develop good posture and proper function.

It's all about finding the right balance between mobility and rigidity. Mobility is often overemphasised when it comes to injury prevention and structural health. Yes, we want to mobilise our joints to relieve excessive muscle tension and allow for good movement. It is, however, essential that our joints have the rigidity to handle the stresses placed on them. This is especially important for your spine.

Mobility is the best place to start, though. As mentioned, it will allow you to relieve any excessive tension and increase your range of motion at various joints, so you can effectively perform the exercises that are designed to increase strength and joint rigidity.

Neck Stretches

The neck is made up of many muscles, and in this section I will show you the most effective stretches for problems in this area.

The deep muscles on the back of the neck

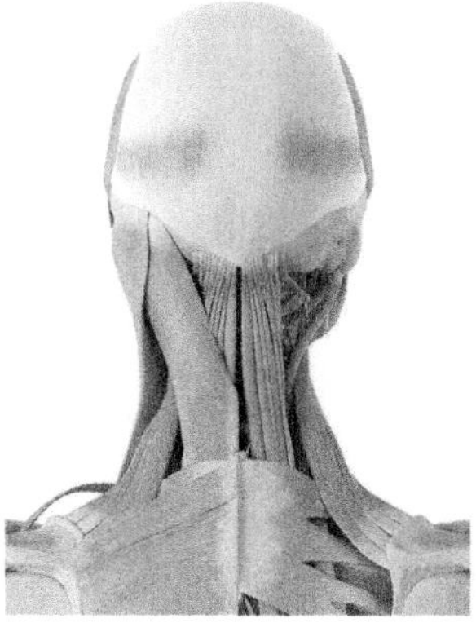

The Levator Scapula

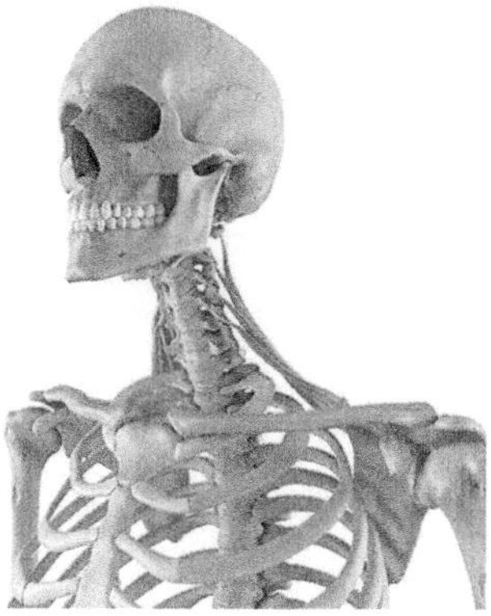

The Trapezius

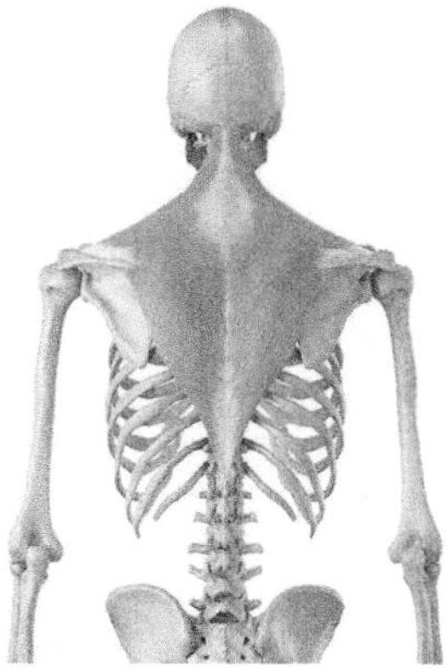

The muscles on the front of your neck

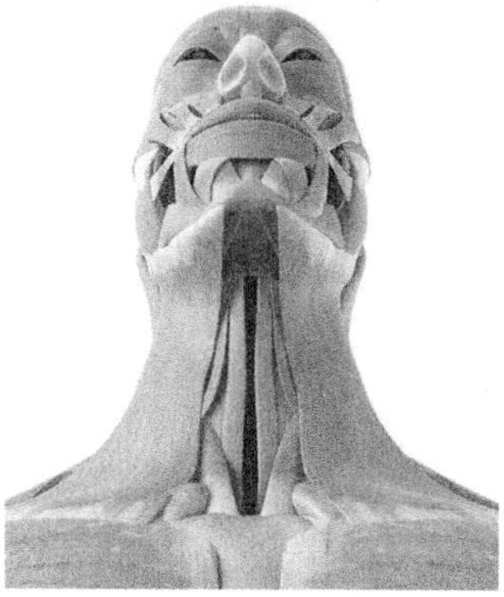

Slow, controlled breathing helps to relax your body and release muscle tension. Taking a deep breath and then slowly exhaling as you increase a stretch is the ideal breathing pattern.

Do not overstretch your neck as you may cause minor strains (these stretches can easily be overdone).

Neck Extensor Stretch:

This stretch is just a small movement, so don't force it. As with any neck stretch, the idea is to stretch the muscles without putting stress on the intervertebral discs.

1. Sit with your chest up and look straight ahead.

2. Gently push your chin back with your hand while looking straight ahead (so that you have a double chin)

3. Keep your head upright, don't look up or down and keep eyes facing forward.

4. While holding your chin back with one hand, use your other hand to reach over the top of your head.

5. Stabilise your chin as you gently pull the top of your head forward and hold a gentle stretch for 20-30 seconds.

6. Complete 1-3 times.

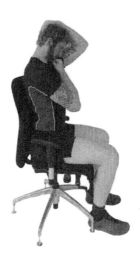

Don't forget; The videos to accompany each exercise are available to download for free from geni.us/fixposture. Simply enrol in the course and you'll have free access to all 34 videos.

Levator Scapula Stretch:

This and the trapezius stretch (next stretch) are quite similar.

If you maintain a forward head posture, the tension in this muscle can be a common source of pain.

1. Sit with your chest up and hold onto the chair with your right hand.

2. Slowly look towards your left pants pocket.

3. Hold the back, right side of your head with your left hand and hold a gentle stretch for 20-30 seconds.

4. To increase the stretch, lean your body slightly towards the left to depress your shoulder further.

5. Repeat on the opposite side.

6. Complete 1-3 times on each side.

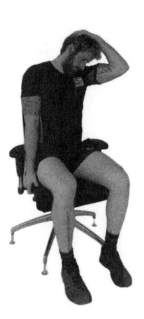

Trapezius Stretch:

Tension in the upper trapezius can cause tension headaches.

1. Sit with your chest up and hold onto the chair with your right hand.

2. Slowly bring your ear towards your left shoulder.

3. Grasp above your right ear with your left hand and hold a gentle stretch for 20-30 seconds

4. To increase the stretch, lean your body slightly towards the left to depress your shoulder further.

5. Repeat on the opposite side.

6. Complete 1-3 times on each side.

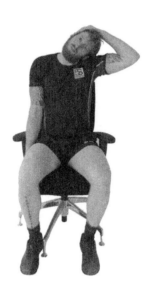

Scalene & Sternocleidomastoid Stretch:

This simple stretch targets the side and the front of your neck.

Tension in the scalene muscles can irritate the nerves that pass through them into the upper extremities, causing problems such as tingling, numbness and pain. Addressing these symptoms is beyond the scope of this book and I recommend you see a specialist to resolve these issues.

Tension in the sternocleidomastoid can also cause pain in your head and face, which this stretch can help relieve.

1. Sit with your chest up and hold onto the chair with your right hand.

2. Rotate your head slightly toward your right.

3. Side bend your head to the left and look upwards as you do so.

4. Hold a gentle stretch for 20-30 seconds.

5. Repeat on the opposite side.

6. Complete 1-3 times on each side.

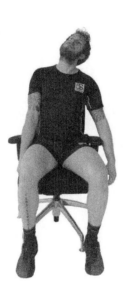

Extra Drill - Trapezius/Neck Release Technique: Barbell Trap Smash!

Here's a great release technique for your trapezius (traps) which can be performed in the gym using a barbell.

A barbell can be utilised as a mobility tool. I have added in a few barbell release techniques throughout the book that can be used to great effect.

1. Set a barbell up on a rack at mid-upper chest height.

2. Place 15kg+ plates on either side.

3. Stand side on to the barbell, bend underneath and push your trapezius up into the barbell.

4. Hold this position for 30-60 seconds and gentle rotate your neck through various movements.

5. During this time, you can also move your left arm through various actions.

6. Repeat on the opposite side.

7. Complete 1-2 times on each side.

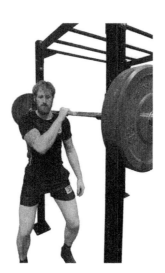

Extra Drill - Trapezius/Neck Release Technique: Barbell Trap Smash!

Chest Release Techniques & Stretches

The musculature of the chest is made up of the pectoralis major and the pectoralis minor (also known as pecs).

These muscles can become tight due to prolonged rounded posture and because people tend to do a lot of pushing actions in day to day life. This can result in an individual not only having rounded shoulders due to bad posture, but tight chest muscles constantly pulling them into this position.

If this is the case, the pectoral group needs to be released and here are some techniques to do so, with variations for at home/office and in the gym.

The Pectoralis Minor   The Pectoralis Major

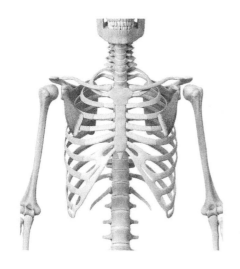
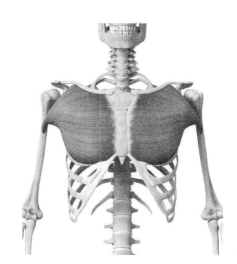

Chest Release Technique:

At home/office:

1. Stand behind a chair.

2. Place your right arm over the back of the chair.

3. Push the soft tissue between your chest and your arm into the top of the chair (just in from your armpit).

4. Hold for 30-60 seconds.

5. Repeat on the opposite side.

6. Complete 1-2 times on each side.

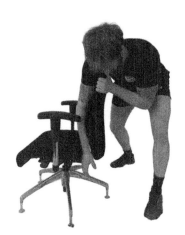

At the gym:

1. Set a barbell up on a rack at hip height.

2. Place your right arm over the barbell.

3. Drive the soft tissue between your chest and your arm into the barbell (just in from your armpit).

4. A weight (dumbbell/kettlebell) can be used to increase the pressure placed on the soft tissues.

5. Slowly move your arm forward and back and in small rotations (with or without weight).

6. Hold for 30-60 seconds.

7. Complete 1-2 times on each side.

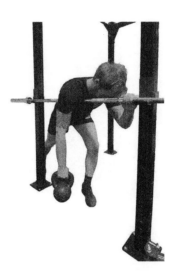

Chest Stretches:

Seated:

This is a simple stretch that can be performed while sitting at your desk.

1. Sit on the front edge of your chair.

2. Clasp your hands together behind your back.

3. Lean forward and raise your hands up behind you.

4. Hold for 30-60 seconds for a regular stretch, or for 2 minutes if the musculature is very tense.

5. Complete 1-3 times.

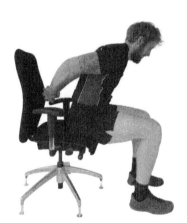

Standing:

This stretch can be performed in a doorway or corner.

1. Raise your hand up with your elbow bent at 90 degrees.

2. Place your forearm along the edge of the door frame/wall and turn your body away from your arm.

3. Hold for 30-60 seconds for a regular stretch, or for 2 minutes if the musculature is very tense.

4. Complete 1-3 times.

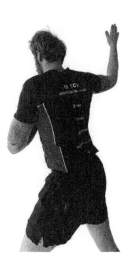

Latissimus Dorsi Release Techniques & Stretches

The latissimus dorsi (lats) is the broadest muscle of the back and is a powerful shoulder extensor, which means it pulls your arms back towards your body from the front or an overhead position.

If this muscle is tight, you will struggle to move your arms overhead and may compensate by arching your lower back, which can lead to back pain.

Tight lats will also negatively affect your shoulder mechanics, pulling your shoulders down as you raise your arms overhead, not allowing for the upwards rotation of your shoulder blades. This can result in shoulder problems such as neck pain and 'impingement', which is when a tendon inside your shoulder rubs or catches on nearby tissue and bone as you lift your arm.

The Latissimus Dorsi

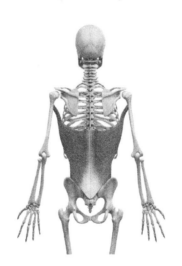

Release Technique - Foam Roller:

1. Sit down on the floor with the foam roller to your right side.

2. Raise your right arm up and lay down on your side, with the foam roller placed onto the latissimus dorsi. You will feel the large muscle mass just below and to the rear of your armpit.

3. Slowly roll up and down the muscle mass for 30-60 seconds.

4. Repeat on the opposite side.

5. Complete 1-2 times on each side.

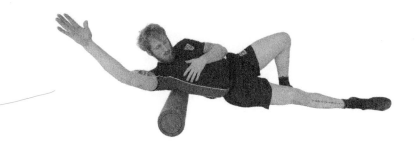

Kneeling Stretch:

This is a simple stretch for your lats which can also be a relaxing position for your hips and lower back.

1. Get onto all fours with your hands placed to your front with your palms flat to the floor.

2. Sit back so your glutes come back towards your heels.

3. Allow your palms to slide forward to facilitate the best stretch. Keep your elbows locked out and spread your fingers.

4. Slowly allow your head to drop between your arms.

5. Hold for 30-60 seconds for a regular stretch, or for 2 minutes if the musculature is very tense.

6. Complete 1-3 times on each side.

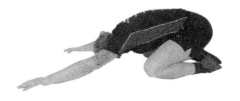

Standing Stretch:

1. Raise your left arm overhead and lean over to your right side. You can bring your right hand up to pull on your left hand slightly.

2. Lean to your right side and forwards while pushing your left hip back. Explore this position to get the best stretch.

3. If you have a something solid such as a doorway, to hold onto with your left hand as you drive your hips back and rotate your back away from the structure it will help to increase the stretch.

4. Hold for 30-60 seconds for a regular stretch, or for 2 minutes if the musculature is very tense.

5. Complete 1-3 times on each side.

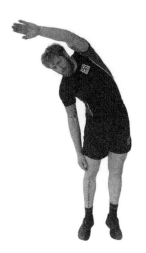 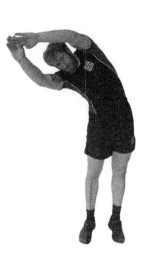

Band Stretch:

This is a great stretch if you have a band and a solid surface to attach it to. It will stretch both your lats and the muscles at the back of your upper arm (triceps).

1. Attach the band to something solid, a vertical or horizontal bar is ideal.

2. Grasp the band with your left hand then turn your back to the band, so your arm is bent over your shoulder with your elbow pointing up towards the ceiling.

3. Step forward with your right leg and lean forward slightly to put tension onto the band.

4. The band tension will pull back on your arm creating a great stretch.

5. Be sure not to lean to far forward, as you could lose balance and injure your arm.

6. Hold for 30-60 seconds for a regular stretch, or for 2 minutes if the musculature is very tense.

7. Complete 1-3 times on each side.

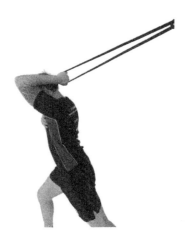

Extra Drill – Wall Angels:

Once you have developed mobility in your lats and pecs, wall angels are a great way to work on shoulder mobility while strengthening the deltoids (shoulders) and traps that facilitate overhead pushing actions.

Although this exercise is simple, it can be quite hard to maintain good form while doing it. I recommend that you develop mobility in your lats and pecs first with the previous stretches before undertaking this exercise.

1. Stand with your back against a wall.

2. Make sure your head, shoulder blades and sacrum (back of pelvis) are flat against the wall.

3. Maintain a natural curve in your lumbar spine. You can flatten your lower back to the wall (posterior pelvic tilt) to help ensure the lats don't pull you into an excessive curve.

4. Place your feet about two foot lengths away from the wall. This will flex your hips and help ensure that your pelvis is kept in a neutral position throughout the movement.

5. Bend your elbows at 90 degrees and place the back of your hands and elbows flat against the wall (as if you're putting your hands up with your elbows bent).

6. While maintaining contact with the wall, slide your hands up the wall until they are in an extended position.

7. Slowly return to the starting position while maintaining contact.

8. Complete 2-4 sets of 5-10 reps.

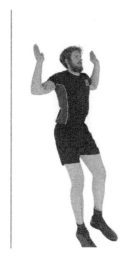 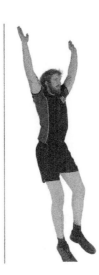

Thoracic Release Techniques

The thoracic spine is the twelve vertebrae between the base of your neck and the bottom of your rib cage. Often when we refer to the thoracic spine in a training environment, we are referring to the muscles which surround it.

The lats are one of the major muscles of the thoracic spine. However, the following drills take a holistic approach to the area, targeting the lats, mid-upper erector spinae, rhomboids, lower-mid traps and pecs, while working to mobilise each individual vertebra.

The back muscles surrounding the Thoracic Spine

The Rhomboids

The Erector Spinae

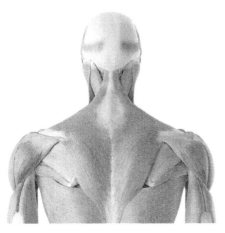
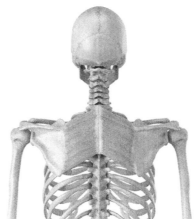
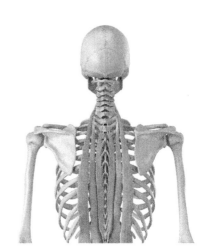

Foam Rolling & Extension Drill:

1. Lie with your mid-back on the foam roller.

2. Extend your arms out in front of you and cross them over each other. You want your shoulders extended to lengthen the muscles of the back.

3. Slowly roll your mid-upper back area up and down for 30-60 seconds.

4. Keep the foam roller static and your arms extended overhead, allowing gravity to do the work and mobilise each vertebra (holding for 30-60 seconds). This is the most effective aspect of foam rolling the thoracic spine.

5. Complete 1-2 times on each side.

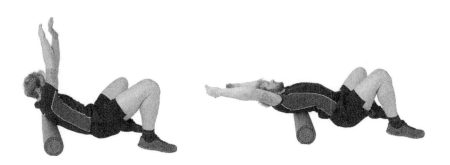

Extra Drill – Barbell Thoracic Extensions:

Use caution when doing this exercise, driving a barbell into the spinous processes, (the bony spur which sticks out from the back of each vertebra), will cause pain and potentially result in injury.

However, when the barbell is placed correctly (just below your shoulder blades), the musculature of your mid-back will cushion the barbell and allow you to perform an effective release technique.

1. Set a barbell up on a rack at mid-thigh height.

2. Crouch down and place your mid-back on the barbell, just below your shoulder blades.

3. Raise your hands overhead. You can do this without weight or with a dumbbell in your hands.

4. Exercise caution with the stretch. If the stretch becomes too much and you can't raise the weight back overhead, simply drop it.

5. Hold the position for 30-60 seconds and allow gravity to do its work.

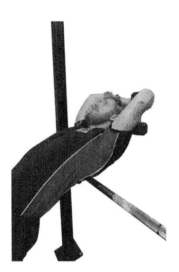

Thoracic Rotations

The lumbar spine has some ability to rotate. However, when performing large rotational actions, your thoracic spine and hips should do most of the work. A great visualisation is to imagine that you are rotating with your chest.

Greater range of motion is achieved when you rotate with both your thoracic spine and hips. However, in this section, we want to isolate thoracic rotation to help mobilise the area.

As mentioned in the posture chapter, during daily activities movement should primarily come from your limbs, with your torso helping to stabilise these actions. If you initiate movements time and time again through bending and rotating your spine, the risk of future back issues is greatly increased.

Seated Stretch:

This is a great stretch to perform at your desk to help free up your upper back.

1. Reach across your body with your left hand and grab under the right side of your seat.

2. Rotate to the right with your thoracic spine and extend your right arm out behind you.

3. Hold the stretch for 30-60 seconds, or for 2 minutes if the musculature is very tense.

4. Complete 1-3 times on each side

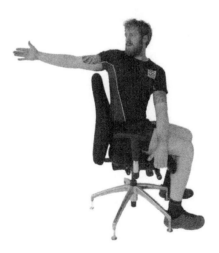

Quadruped Thoracic Rotations:

This is a great stretch for mobilising your upper back. However, it can make you feel a little dizzy so take care when standing afterwards.

1. Get down onto all fours.

2. Place your left hand behind your head.

3. Shifting back with your hips facilitates a small degree of lumbar flexion, which will take away the arch. This ensures you don't compensate for the movement by rotating your lumbar spine.

4. Place your left elbow under your torso before rotating round and pointing it toward the ceiling, or as far as your mobility will allow.

5. Follow your elbow with your eyes.

6. Complete 2-3 sets of 5-10 rotations on each side.

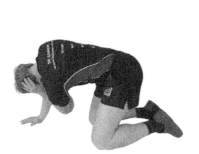 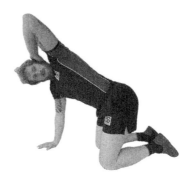

Side Lying Thoracic Rotations:

1. Lay on your side.

2. Raise the top leg up to 90 degrees, resting it on a foam roller.

3. Place your hands out to the front in a prayer position.

4. Slowly rotate with your thoracic spine to bring the top arm over so that the back of your hand touches the floor, or as far as mobility allows.

5. Keep your leg firmly on the foam roller throughout the whole movement.

6. Complete 2-3 sets of 5-10 rotations on each side.

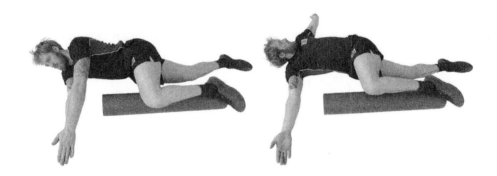

Chapter 4: Shoulder External Rotation & Retraction Strength

Introduction

Now that I have shown you various techniques for regaining and maintaining mobility in your upper body, it is time to look at how to strengthen associated muscles to help reinforce optimal posture.

The chances of you achieving perfect symmetry in every muscle group is slim because, for example, your right arm may be stronger at certain actions than your left and vice versa. However, you should work towards gaining the best symmetry you can.

The first exercises in this chapter are very basic and work on small, specific movements. They are followed by compound exercises which work multiple joints and muscle groups to achieve a greater overall effect.

While it's beneficial to work on specific muscles that may need extra attention, it is also essential that you work large combined movements. After all, the body works as one big kinetic chain, not as individual muscles performing tasks independently.

Head Retractions & Scapula Pinches

Forward head posture can result in tension headaches, and upper back and neck pain.

Head retractions will build a certain degree of strength, especially if resistance is used. However, the main benefit of this exercise is that it helps to build your awareness of proper head positioning. Practise often and it will help to ingrain correct posture.

Head Retractions:

1. Sit upright in your chair.

2. Pull your chin back and slightly up. A tip for getting this right is to place your finger on the vertical groove between your upper lip and nose (your philtrum), push softly and allow your head to retract.

3. Hold the position for 3-5 seconds before releasing.

4. Complete 3-5 sets of 5-10 reps throughout the day.

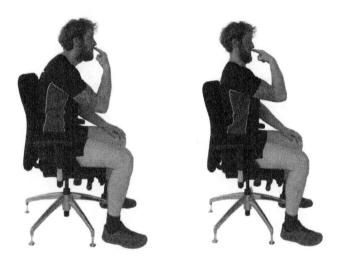

Don't forget; The videos to accompany each exercise are available to download for free from geni.us/fixposture. Simply enrol in the course and you'll have free access to all 34 videos.

Scapula Pinches:

Scapula (shoulder blade) pinches are a great exercise. Not only do they free up your upper back, they work to strengthen the muscles which retract your shoulder blades. They can be done while standing or seated.

1. Stand/sit with good posture, relax your shoulders and extend them forward slightly.

2. Pull your shoulders back and concentrate on squeezing your shoulder blades together. Feel your lower traps and rhomboids (muscles between your shoulder blades) scrunch up.

3. H old the position for 3-5 seconds.

4. Release and slowly bring your shoulders forward.

5. Complete 3-5 sets of 5-10 reps.

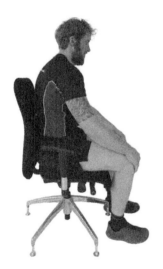 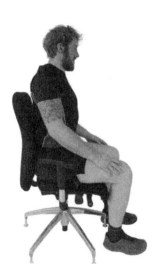

Extra Drill - Seated Shoulder Rolls:

Seated shoulder rolls are an easy exercise that you can do every 30-40 minutes while sitting at your desk. They help to mobilise your shoulders and free up tension.

I recommend adding a set of these in before and after your head retractions and scapula pinches.

1. Sit upright in good posture, ensure you chin is back.

2. Raise your right shoulder up towards your ear and roll it back.

3. Do the same with your left shoulder.

4. Complete 1-2 sets of 5-10 rotations on each side.

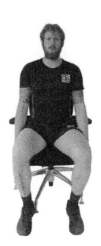 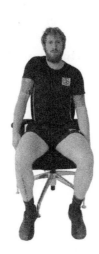 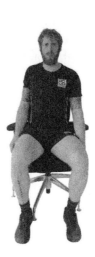

Shoulder External Rotation

If someone has a slouched upper body posture with rounded shoulders, their shoulders are often internally rotated. That is, their hands are rotated inwards so that their palms are facing behind them.

The rotator cuff is four deep muscles responsible for stabilising the shoulder joint, as well as both internal and external rotation (rotating the hands back out so the palms are facing forward). One muscle works as an internal rotator, while the other three work to externally rotate the shoulders.

The internal rotator, along with your chest muscles, often gets plenty of work (due to lots of pushing actions), whereas your external rotators are often underworked, which can result in postural issues.

It's these postural issues that can cause all sorts of problems when you start to bench press and overhead press at the gym. People often say, "the bench press is bad for your shoulders", but in actuality, it's poor posture and poor lifting mechanics/technique on the bench that is bad for your shoulders.

It's vital that we work muscles in a way that specifically target their different roles. The rotator cuff primarily works to stabilise the shoulder joint as it performs various actions. Although facilitating repeated external rotations may not be its main role, all muscles benefit from having their secondary and tertiary actions worked. This exercise will create a deep burn in your shoulders!

The Supraspinatus – One of the rotator cuffs

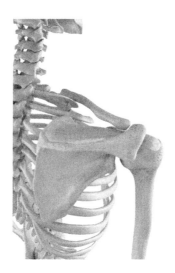

External Rotations – Long Band:

1. Attach a long band to something solid at abdominal height. Use a yellow or red band, increasing tension by standing further from the attachment point if required.

2. Grasp the band with your right hand and turn side on so that your left shoulder is closest to the attachment point.

3. Stand with good posture, bend your right elbow to 90 degrees and keep it tucked into your side.

4. Pull the band across your body while externally rotating your right shoulder. Ensure your body stays forward facing and your right elbow remains tucked into your side.

5. Once you have reached the limit of your range of motion with your elbow tucked in, slowly return to the starting position.

6. Don't allow the band to jerk you back to the starting position. Keep it controlled throughout the whole movement.

7. If your elbow comes away from your side, your large shoulder muscle (delt) will take over, so it's important to hold it close.

8. Complete 2-4 sets of 10 reps on each side.

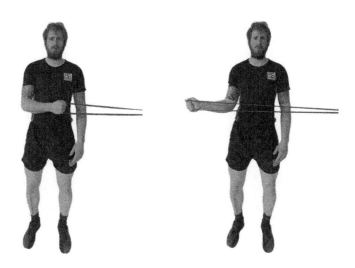

External Rotations – Small Loop Band:

1. Small loop bands come in varying colours. For this exercise, you will need a low-tension band.

2. Hold the band with both hands. I usually place my thumbs over the band.

3. Bend your elbows at 90 degrees and keep both elbows tucked into your sides.

4. Externally rotate both shoulders at the same time.

5. Don't allow the band to jerk you back to the starting position. Keep it controlled throughout the whole movement.

6. Complete 2-4 sets of 10 reps

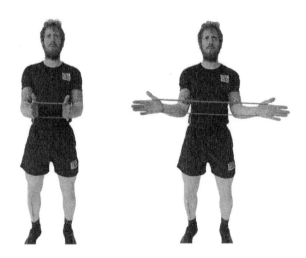

Serratus Wall Slides

Wall slides are a great exercise for your serratus anterior, which is often referred to as the 'boxer's muscle' due to its job in protracting your shoulders (reaching forward), an action used when you throw a punch.

The serratus anterior muscle originates on the underside of each shoulder blade and wraps around the rib cage (often visible as a jagged muscle on well trained individuals). These muscles work to pull your shoulder blades flat to your ribcage, while pulling them away from the spine. They aid the upward rotation of your shoulder blades along with your traps.

Upwards rotation is essential for maintaining shoulder health while throwing or pushing your arms overhead. If your shoulder blades don't rotate upwards you're at far greater risk of impingement (rubbing of a tendon) in your shoulders.

If you imagine your shoulder blades being held down while you try to take your arms overhead, you can feel how motion of the shoulder blades is vital for achieving overhead positions.

The Serratus Anterior

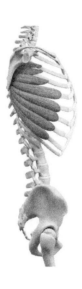

Serratus Wall Slides – Foam Roller:

This exercise uses a foam roller to facilitate the movement smoothly.

1. Place the roller against a wall.

2. Facing the wall/foam roller, bend your elbows to 90 degrees and place your forearms on the roller, with the roller just below your wrists.

3. Drive your forearms into the roller as if you are pushing yourself away, extending your shoulders and engaging the serratus.

4. Keep your head back and roll the roller up so that your shoulders flex and your elbows start to extend.

5. Feel your serratus engage and roll until the roller meets your elbow. Imagine the bottom of your shoulder blades rotating outwards and upwards towards your armpit.

6. Relax as you roll back down to the starting position.

7. Complete 2-4 sets of 5-10 reps.

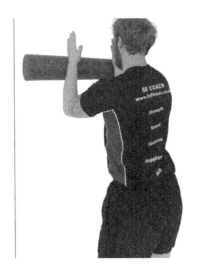 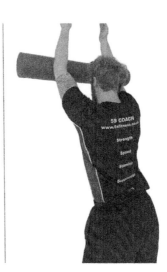

Band Pull Apart

As a strength and conditioning coach who works with athletes and the general public, I can't overstate how effective band pull apart variations are at restoring and maintaining shoulder health. Every one of the clients I have prescribed these to has had amazing results.

Band pull apart variations are especially great for lifters, but any individual who is looking to restore and maintain good upper-body posture and shoulder health will benefit from them.

During these exercises it's important not to shrug your shoulders and bring your upper traps into play. You want to work the musculature of the upper back that is responsible for shoulder retraction, not elevation.

Standard Pull Apart:

1. Use a yellow or red long band. The tension can be varied by taking a wider or narrower grip.

2. Take an overhand grip (palms facing down) on the band and place your arms out in front of you with your elbows straight. Grip the band at shoulder width if you can.

3. With your arms straight, pull your arms outwards so the band stretches and comes to your mid chest.

4. The band can also be pulled to your abdomen or forehead to vary the angle at which your shoulders are working.

5. Don't allow the band to jerk you back to the starting position. Keep it under control throughout the whole movement.

6. Complete 2-4 sets of 10-20 reps.

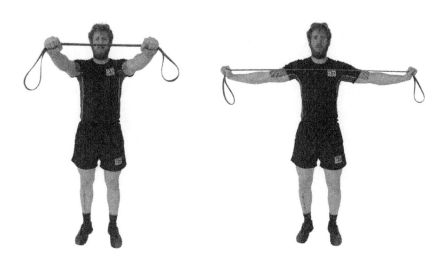

Star Pattern:

The star pattern pull apart is a variation which cycles through various pulling positions.

1. Start with the standard pull apart to your mid chest.

2. Pull your right hand downwards and your left arm upwards so the band comes diagonally across your body.

3. Repeat this action but the opposite way around, right hand upwards and left hand downwards.

4. Repeat the standard pull apart to your upper chest to restart the cycle.

5. Complete 2-4 sets of 10-20 reps (each pull apart = 1 rep).

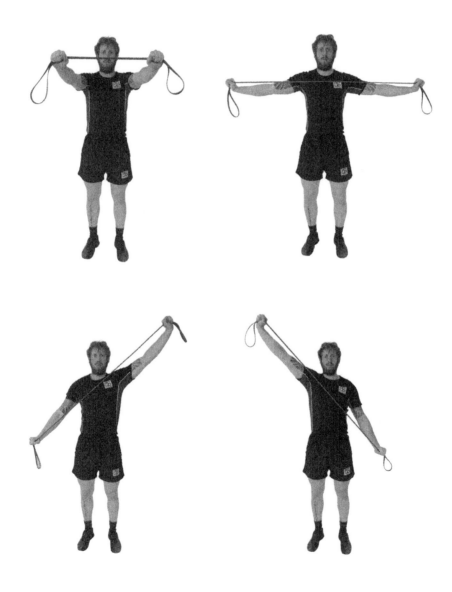

Extra Drill – Band Front-to-Backs:

The band front-to-back is a great mobility drill for your shoulders that can be practised anytime. I am placing it here with the band pull apart variations as they work well together.

The pull apart works the muscles that retract your shoulders; the front-to-back mobilises all the muscles that restrict shoulder retraction and overhead positions, such as pecs.

1. Grab a red band with a wide overhand grip. The wider your arms, the easier it is to take the band overhead and down towards your glutes.

2. The band allows you the freedom to widen your grip as you pass it overhead. Your grip should be wide enough so that you aren't forced to aggressively stretch the band out as you perform the movement, as this can cause you to shrug your shoulders, engaging musculature rather than promoting mobility.

3. Start with the band at your hips and while maintaining straight arms throughout, pass it overhead until it reaches your glutes, or the range of motion you can achieve.

4. Complete 2-4 sets of 5-10 reps.

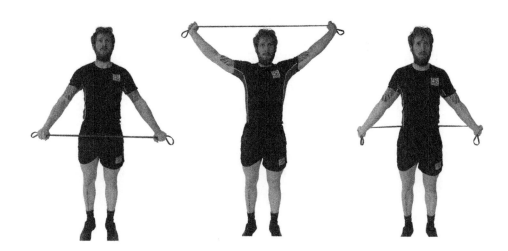

Band Face Pulls

Face pulls are one of the best exercises to rehabilitate and develop your upper back and shoulders.

Resistance bands apply 'accommodating resistance', so the resistance will increase as you progress through the exercise. This helps to maximise the contraction of the muscles at work, as you get to the top of the face pull, your rear delts, traps and rhomboids are going to have to increase their engagement to overcome the extra resistance as the band tension increases.

1. Use a yellow or red band. You can vary the tension by standing closer or further away from the band attachment point.

2. Attach the band to something solid at chest height, either looping the band around and holding both ends, or looping the band through itself so you have hold of one end of the band with both hands.

3. Facing the attachment point, grab the band with an overhand grip. You can grasp the band with just your fingers rather than taking a full grip. This will help to encourage the upper back to work as the primary mover rather than the biceps.

4. Step backwards to apply tension to the band.

5. Keep your chin back.

6. Pull backwards and slightly up to bring yourself into a double bicep pose position. Maintain good head posture, pull your hands back to your temples and don't push your head towards the band.

7. Ensure you consciously engage your upper back and rear delts, rather than just pulling with your biceps – think about the muscle you are working to increase its engagement (mind-muscle connection).

8. Return to the starting position under control, allowing your shoulders to extend slightly.

9. Complete 2-4 sets of 10-20 reps.

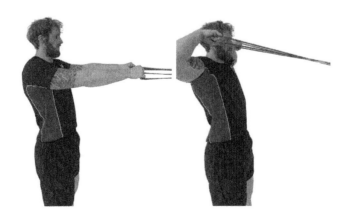

Band Horizontal Pulls

Horizontal pulling actions can be done well on cable/resistance machines. However, bands are more accessible and have the added benefit of accommodating resistance.

I recommend you incorporate horizontal pulling exercises as much as you can. It's commonly recommended for those that train often to incorporate 2-3 times more pulling than pushing.

Bilateral:

Bilateral refers to using both sides of your body at the same time. This exercise can be done while standing or sitting.

1. Use a red or higher tension band. The tension can be varied by standing closer or further away from the band attachment point.

2. Attach the band to something solid at abdominal/lower chest height. Facing the attachment point, grab each end of the band with a neutral grip.

3. Walk backwards to apply tension to the band.

4. Pull the band to your sides, ensuring you consciously engage your back muscles, rather than just pulling with your biceps (mind-muscle connection).

5. Ensure you really concentrate on retracting your shoulders

6. Return to the starting position under control, allowing your shoulders to protract slightly.

7. Complete 2-4 sets of 10-20 reps.

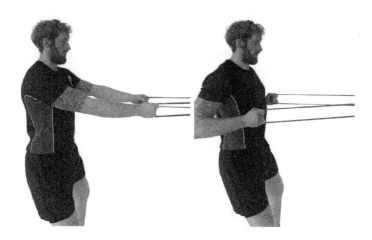

Unilateral:

The unilateral pull involves the same set up as the bilateral pull, but both ends of the band are held in one hand.

The unilateral pull works as a great anti-rotation exercise (discussed in more detail in chapter six). This is essentially a core exercise which works the muscles that resist rotational forces on your spine, which are integral for injury prevention.

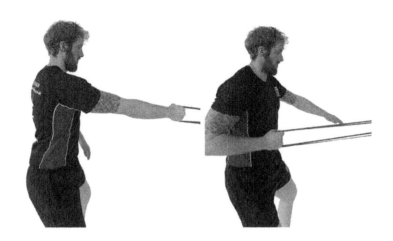

Bent Over Rows

The final few exercises can be done with a band, or small dumbbells if you have them available. You can even use improvised equipment such as cans of food. However, this section of the chapter is geared towards working with heavier loads for greater strength development.

It's important that you build strength and endurance in the small muscles that support you as these can often be the cause of various issues. However, you also need to develop proper movement. All the smaller and more specific drills in this book should ultimately progress you to larger movements which work various joints and muscle groups in unison rather than isolation.

Your body is only going to adapt if it is stressed to a point that warrants adaptation. When it comes to the development of strength, increasing the stress by increasing the load is the best way to get improvements.

Although strength is often simply defined as the highest amount of force you can exert to overcome a resistance (usually in a single effort). It is also about the robustness of the interconnected systems that make up your structure; your skeletal system and soft tissues.

Strength is the foundation of all physical aspects of life. If you lack the ability to accommodate the stresses placed on your body, you will potentially be full of aches and pains.

The barbell is the most efficient tool for total strength development. You can squat, push, and pull (three major strength movements) a barbell and increase the weight over weeks and months, progressively loading your muscles with more and more weight, which is the key to any decent training programme. The bent over row can also be performed with a resistance band (pictured below).

When considering what weight to use, start with 1-2 warm up sets to get a feel for the movement, prior to selecting a weight that should ideally have you struggling on the last 2 or 3 reps.

The bent over row is a great exercise that works the musculature of your back and your biceps. It is essentially the bilateral horizontal band pull performed from a standing, bent over position, and works the muscles in the same way.

I recommend starting with an overhand grip. An underhand grip can be used and works the mid-back and biceps. However, the overhand grip is by far the most commonly used grip when working with a barbell and it is often the default grip for heavy rows. Work with both variants and see which works best for you.

1. Pick the barbell up, ensuring you use proper technique to do so.

2. Hinge at your hips by pushing your glutes back and allowing your torso to drop forward.

3. As you hinge, bend your knees slightly to bring the barbell to your knee or slightly below (this depends on limb length).

4. Your back position should be midway between standing straight up, and bending double at the waist (see picture).

5. Pull the barbell up to just above your navel and control it as it lowers back down to the starting position, allowing your shoulders to protract slightly to stretch the muscles of your back.

6. Complete 3-5 sets of 5-10 reps.

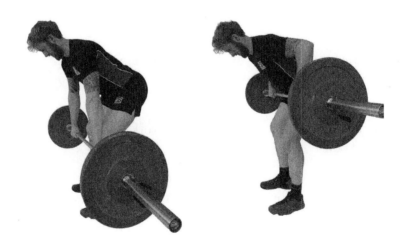

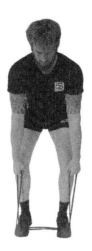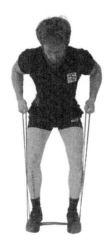

Single Arm Rows

Bilateral movements that work both sides of the body simultaneously such as the bent over row are integral for strength development. However, unilateral exercises such as the single arm row also have many benefits.

The single arm row is essentially the unilateral horizontal band pull performed from a standing, bent over position.

The single arm row can be performed with a resistance band (pictured below). However, I will be explaining the dumbbell variation in more detail as you will see greater benefit from progressively adding weight to this movement.

Using a single dumbbell allows you to facilitate more rotation through your upper back during the row, which in turn allows for a greater stretch on your lats. Maximising the range of motion and facilitating a good stretch of the muscle prior to it contracting and pulling the weight up increases the intensity of the exercise.

Performing bent over rows with the weight on one side also works as a great anti-rotation exercise, just like the unilateral horizontal band pulls.

1. Single arm rows can be done with the knee and hand on the same side supported on a bench, or with just one hand on a bench as support. I personally prefer a single hand support.

2. For the single hand supported row, hinge at your hips and bend your knees slightly, placing your right hand on the bench.

3. Your feet should be slightly wider than shoulder width apart, either side by side or in a 'split stance' where the same leg of the arm rowing is behind you.

4. Rows can be done with your torso parallel to the floor. However, a position where your shoulders are slightly higher than your hips will work the upper back more.

5. Bend your knees to pick up the dumbbell before raising it up 5-10 inches off the floor.

6. Pull the dumbbell up to your side, ensuring you consciously engage your back and rear delts to retract your shoulders.

7. Lower the dumbbell, keeping it under control, and allow your shoulders to protract slightly to stretch the muscles of your back.

8. Complete 3-5 sets of 8-15 reps on each side.

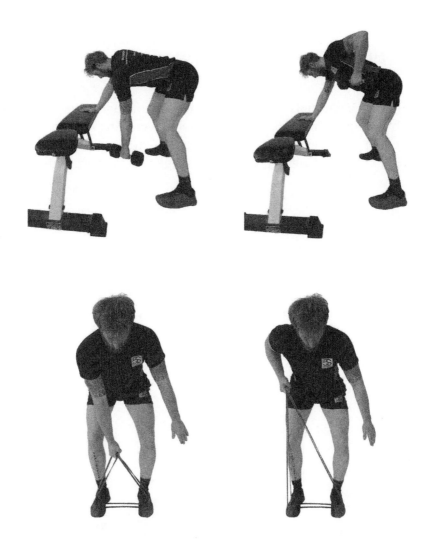

Bent Over Lateral Raises

Bent over lateral raises are sometimes referred to as 'rear flys', and are a great postural exercise.

I recommend using moderate weight for this exercise as overloading can result in you jerking the dumbbells up, instead of using a controlled movement.

Having a slight jerking action when lifting heavy weight is not always a terrible thing, sometimes we simply want to move a heavy weight from point A to point B in order to make strength gains. However, the aim of these exercises is to concentrate on working the muscles which retract your shoulders. This needs to be done in a smooth movement.

The 'pitcher method' is often used during lateral raise variations with dumbbells. This involves turning your thumbs down as you reach the top of the movement (as if you are pouring out a pitcher). This method does help to get more engagement of your rear delts. However, it also increases the risk of shoulder impingement. Instead, use a slight hinge of your hips while performing upright lateral raises, and finish in the bent over position to hit your rear delts.

1. Holding a dumbbell in each hand, hinge at your hips, allowing your torso to drop forward as in the bent over row (an angle of 45-60 degrees). Keep your chin tucked in.

2. Allow the dumbbells to drop to your front and hold them together, creating a slight bend in your elbows. This bend remains throughout the lift.

3. Raise your arms out to the side, concentrating on retracting your shoulder blades and really working your rear delts and rhomboids (muscles between your shoulder blades).

4. Return to the starting position.

5. Complete 3-5 sets of 8-15 reps.

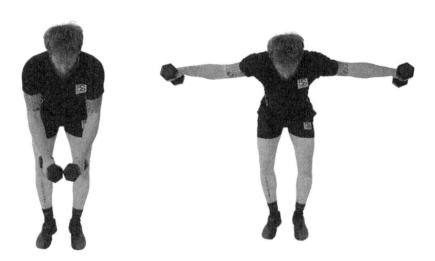

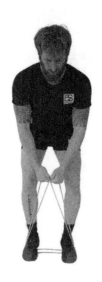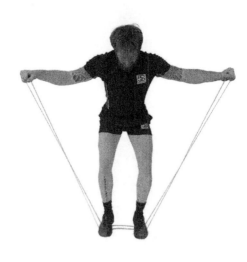

Shrugs

Shrugs work shoulder elevation by raising your shoulders up towards your ears. We want to train the upper traps to keep them in good health.

Having one shoulder higher than the other is very common, often due to the way you stand/sit, or which hand you tend to carry stuff in.

Although varying shoulder heights can stem from the spine or pelvis, it's not difficult to look in the mirror and see if one trap is a little more developed and pulling the shoulder higher, while the other is undeveloped and slack. If you have one shoulder higher than the other, a simple fix is to perform single arm shrugs on the side that is under developed, while stretching the other side.

For overall development of the traps, simply shrug with dumbbells in both hands or, if you have access to one, use a hex bar - a specialist barbell which is designed perfectly for shrugging actions.

The shrug can also be performed with a resistance band (pictured below). Simply stand upright on the resistance band, with the band in each hand and shrug.

1. Stand upright in good posture with a dumbbell in each hand at your sides.

2. Brace your core.

3. With straight arms, shrug your shoulder upwards as high as you can. Don't use a circular motion, simply move up and down.

4. Ensure your shoulders are driving upwards and you are not driving your head downwards.

5. Try to inhale during the effort/upwards phase of the lift, rather than during the downward phase (opposite to most strength exercises).

6. Hold at the top for a second or two before slowly lowering the dumbbells back down to the starting position.

7. Complete 3-5 sets of 8-15 reps.

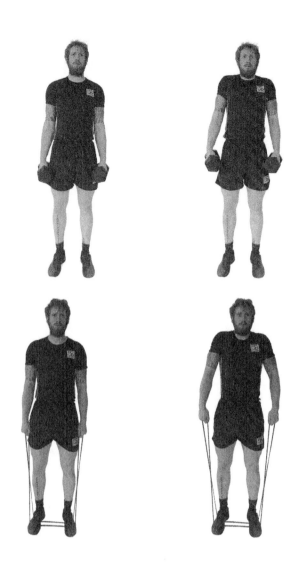

Chapter 5: Hip & Core Mobility

Introduction

Now we have looked at how you can regain and maintain both mobility and strength in the upper body. We will do the same for your lower body, focussing on your hips and core.

Your core is the musculature of your torso, but more specifically it is the lumbo-pelvic region (lumbar spine and pelvis, often referred to as your 'low back'). These muscles are responsible for both stabilisation and the transfer of force from one aspect of movement to the next, for example changing direction.

The lumbo-pelvic region is really at the heart of good movement and if there are any postural issues, muscular imbalances, or weaknesses in this area, it can cause problems that can manifest themselves from head to toe.

In this chapter, I will be showing you release techniques and stretches for the major muscle groups that surround your hips, specifically those that can become problematic due to prolonged sitting.

Hip Flexor/Quadriceps Release Techniques & Stretches

Your hip flexors do exactly what you'd expect: flex your hips. Prolonged sitting leaves your hip flexors in a shortened position, often resulting in them becoming tense.

Since one of the hip flexors (psoas major) originates on your lower spine while the other originates on your pelvis (iliacus), they can pull on your lower spine, putting your hips into an anterior tilt, often resulting in back pain.

Your quadriceps (thighs) can also play a role with tightness in this area, as one of the quads also acts as a hip flexor (rectus femoris). So, it is beneficial to also roll the quads with a foam roller.

The Iliacus:
One of the hip flexors

The Psoas Major:
One of the hip flexors

The Rectus Femoris:
A quadricep muscle that also
acts as a hip flexor

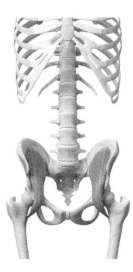

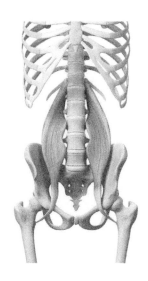

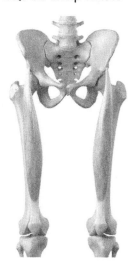

Release Technique – Foam Roller or Massage Ball:

The deep origin of the hip flexors mean that you are not going to be able to get a great deal of self-myofascial release to the area. However, you can target some of the more superficial tissue that crosses your hip joint.

You can also foam roll right down to your knee to release your quads while in this position.

1. Place the foam roller or massage ball on the floor.

2. Lay onto the roller at the crease of your hip on one side. Practise caution when placing a massage ball into the crease of the hip or groin area to not overly stress the area.

3. Slowly roll up and down the muscle mass for 30-60 seconds.

4. Complete 1-2 sets on each side.

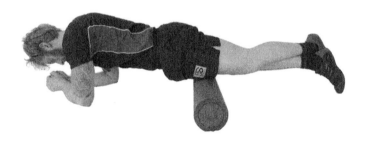

Hip Flexor Stretches:

Kneeling:

The hip flexors are an easy muscle to stretch. However, individuals often adopt a position that throws their pelvis into an anterior tilt. This can exacerbate any low back pain they may be suffering from. It's far more effective to keep your pelvis in a neutral position while squeezing your glutes.

Often, we can get one muscle set to relax by squeezing an opposing muscle set, known as 'reciprocal inhibition'. Contracting the glutes helps to facilitate a greater stretch.

1. Adopt a half kneeling position, your left knee down and your right foot flat on the floor to the front, with a knee bend of 90 degrees.

2. Squeeze your glutes, focussing on the left side, and drive your left hip forward into hyperextension to facilitate the stretch. Your pelvis should remain neutral throughout.

3. Raising the same arm to the hip flexor you are stretching and reaching over the opposite shoulder really increases the stretch through the hip flexors and the quads.

4. Hold for 30-60 seconds, or for 2 minutes if the musculature is very tense.

5. Complete 1-3 times on each side.

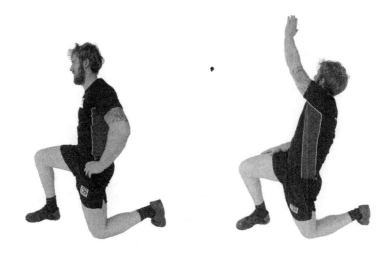

Couch:

The couch stretch is an effective variation that can increase the intensity of both the hip flexor and quad stretch.

The stretch can be done with the leg being stretched up behind you against a wall or with the upper side of the foot placed on a bench or chair, allowing your knee to rest on the floor or a well cushioned mat.

1. Place your right leg against a wall or the top of your foot onto a raised platform which is just below knee height.

2. This places you in a half kneeling position with your left foot flat on the floor to the front with a knee bend of 90 degrees.

3. Squeeze your glutes, specifically the right side and drive your right hip forward into hyper-extension to facilitate the stretch. Your pelvis should remain neutral.

4. Raising the arm on the side of the stretch, and reaching over the opposite shoulder increases the stretch.

5. Hold for 30-60 seconds, or for 2 minutes if the musculature is very tense.

6. Complete 1-3 times on each side.

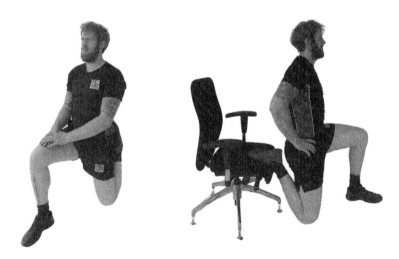

Glute/Piriformis Release Techniques & Stretches

The three muscles of the glutes are often considered to be an area that needs extra attention when it comes to strength. However, they often become tense, causing pain in your low back and hamstrings.

The piriformis is a small muscle that is located under your main buttock muscle (gluteus maximus). The sciatic nerve travels either underneath or through the piriformis.

The Gluteus Maximus

The Piriformis

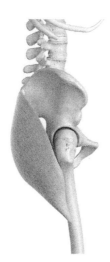
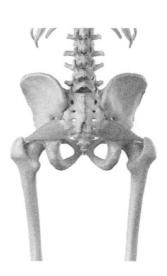

Release Technique – Foam Roller or Massage Ball:

You must be very careful with the glutes when attempting self-myofascial release. This is due to the location of the sciatic nerve which passes through the gluteal area and down your leg.

Driving a massage ball into your sciatic nerve is potentially going to leave you with worse symptoms than those you are trying to relieve. It is essential that you target the musculature on the upper gluteal area only.

I do not recommend using release techniques on this area if you are suffering from sciatic pain, or are not completely confident on how you can safely work the soft tissues.

1. Place a foam roller or massage ball on the floor. A foam roller will help to distribute the pressure across the gluteal area and so will be less intense.

2. Sit on the roller with your upper gluteal area (where your back pockets would be).

3. To roll your right side, place your right leg over your left so the ankle of your right leg is just above your left knee. This lengthens the musculature being worked.

4. If this is not possible, simply drop your right knee off to the side.

5. Slowly roll up and down the muscle mass for 30-60 seconds.

6. Complete 1-2 times on each side.

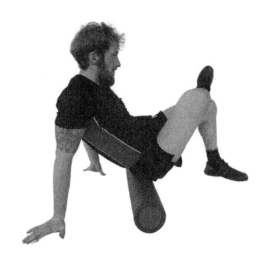

Glute Stretches:

Seated:

This stretch for your glutes and piriformis can easily be facilitated at your desk.

1. Sit upright in your chair.

2. To stretch your right side, place your right leg over your left so the ankle of your right leg is just above your left knee.

3. Keeping your chest proud, lean towards your right knee. Don't round your spine and bend your head down towards your knee, push your chest forward with a neutral spine.

4. Hold for 30-60 seconds, or for 2 minutes if the musculature is very tense.

5. Complete 1-3 times on each side.

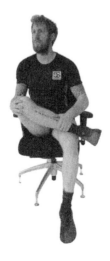

Figure Four:

1. Lie on your back.

2. To stretch your right side, raise your left leg up with your knee bent at 90 degrees.

3. Place your right leg over your left so the ankle of your right leg is just below your left knee.

4. Reach through and grab round the back of your left leg with both hand and pull towards your chest.

5. Hold for 30-60 seconds, or for 2 minutes if the musculature is very tense.

6. Complete 1-3 times on each side.

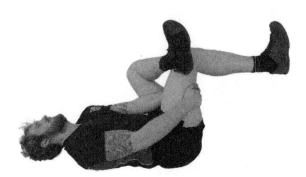

Pigeon Stretch:

1. Start on all fours.

2. To stretch your right side, place the outer side of your right leg onto the floor. The sole of your right foot will be pointing to the left while your knee is pointing to the right.

3. Slide your left leg back as you move your right leg into position.

4. Keep your hips forward-facing and your chest proud, driving your chest upwards to increase the stretch.

5. If you can, keep your right foot in line with your right knee. However, you might need to pull your foot back towards your hip.

6. Hold for 30-60 seconds, or for 2 minutes if the musculature is very tense.

7. Complete 1-3 times on each side.

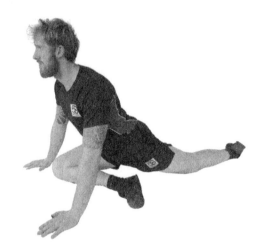

Low Back Release Techniques & Stretches

The muscles of the lower back can often become tense and this can cause low back pain.

A major culprit of this pain is often the quadratus lumborum (QL) and/or lower erector spinae. These muscles are located on either side of the spine and attach to your pelvis, so any imbalances can cause postural issues which have negative effects on your whole body.

I don't recommend rolling the lower back with a long foam roller. Unlike the thoracic spine, the lumbar spine is not surrounded by other skeletal structures such as your rib cage and shoulder blades, which help support the area. Although the thoracic spine often benefits from extension drills on the roller, your lumbar spine may not. Often driving a roller into your lower spine will simply cause your lower back muscles to tighten, as they try to protect your spine.

I prefer to work each side of the spine independently with a massage ball, either laying on it, or placing it on a wall or a door frame so I can also push back against the other side.

The Quadratus Lumborum

The Erector Spinae

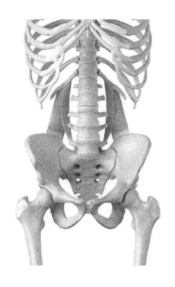 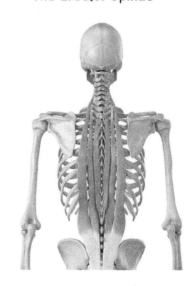

Release Techniques – Massage Ball:

You can buy massage balls that are a peanut shape so you can work both sides without applying pressure to the vertebra. However, I feel you can get much deeper when using a single massage ball on one side.

1. Place the ball on the floor if lying on it, or against a wall or door frame at hip height.

2. Place the right side of your lower back onto the ball, just above your pelvis.

3. Keep your pelvis neutral or tilted slightly backwards to drive the soft tissue into the ball.

4. If lying, you can raise the knee of the side you are working, to allow you to drive the ball deeper into the soft tissue.

5. If working in a door frame or similar space, you can push against the structure to the front of you to increase the depth.

6. Slowly roll up and down the muscle mass for 30-60 seconds.

7. Complete 1-2 times on each side.

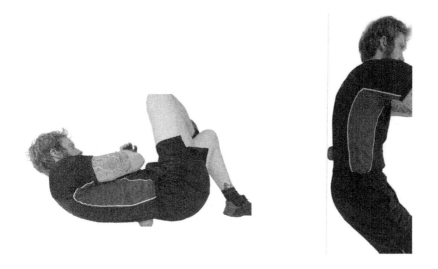

Hip Rolls:

This is a simple exercise that will help to mobilise your lower back.

A useful stretch that can be coupled with this exercise is to bring one or both knees to your chest in the lying position. This will stretch your lower back, glutes and hamstrings.

1. Lie on your back with your head flat to the floor and your arms spread to your sides.

2. Bend your knees so your soles are flat on the floor.

3. Slowly roll your knees side to side while keeping both arms flat to the floor.

4. Complete 2-3 sets of 10-20 rolls.

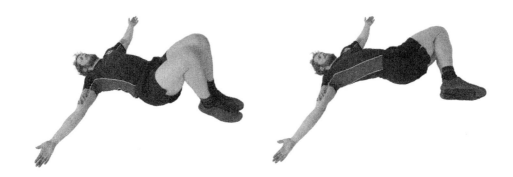

Iron Cross Stretch:

The iron cross stretch mobilises your hips and lower back, and acts as a great warm up drill.

1. Lie on your back with your head flat to the floor and your arms spread to your sides.

2. While keeping the other leg flat to the floor, slowly raise one leg and bring it towards your opposite hand.

3. Hold this position for 2-3 seconds before returning it to the starting position and proceeding with the opposite leg.

4. Complete 2-3 sets of 10 reps.

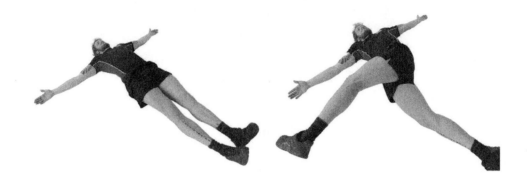

Rectus Abdominis & Oblique Stretches

Your anterior core musculature (abdominals) tends to get a lot of attention due to their importance aesthetically.

Although it's important for these muscles to be strong, they can become excessively tense due to getting plenty of training without much stretching. This is often reinforced by prolonged sitting in a hunched posture that leaves them in a shortened position.

Both the rectus abdominis (6-pack muscles) and the obliques (musculature to the side of the 6-pack) all attach between your ribs and your pelvis, and any muscle mass that attaches to your pelvis can influence pelvic positioning and have a role in ailments such as low back pain.

Earlier, I discussed the importance of thoracic mobility and how to specifically target the area to ensure good posture and shoulder health. If your abdominal muscles are tight and pulling your rib cage closer to your pelvis, then this is also going to affect your ability to extend your thoracic spine. So, this is an area that needs to be considered when trying to rectify thoracic mobility issues.

The Rectus Abdominis   The External Obliques

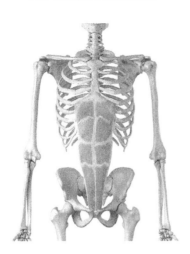
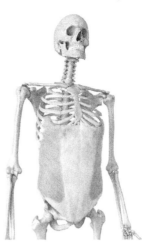

Lying Abdominal Stretch:

This is often referred to as a 'cobra stretch' due to the way you are curled up from the floor. Although it is a helpful stretch, caution must be practised as your lower spine will be hyperextended. If you suffer with extension-based back pain, this is not a stretch for you.

To test whether your back pain is extension-based or flexion-based, a basic cat camel drill can be used.

To perform the cat camel, adopt a quadruped position and simply round (flex) and dip (extend) your spine. If the extended position exacerbates your back pain then you are suffering with extension-based back pain, if the flexed position exacerbates your back pain, then you are suffering with flexion-based pain.

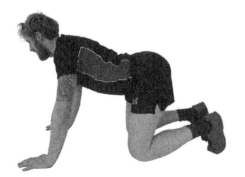
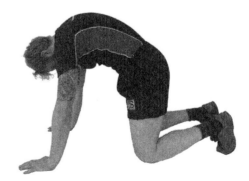

Individuals that suffer with extension-based back pain will often get into a kneeling lat stretch or lie on their back and bring their knees to their chest to alleviate discomfort, both of which put the lower spine into a flexed (rounded) position.

Individuals that suffer with flexion-based back pain often place their hands on their hips and hyperextend their spine, or adopt the following cobra position to alleviate discomfort.

1. Lie on your stomach.

2. While keeping your hips on the floor use your forearms or hands to raise your torso up.

3. You will be hyperextending through your spine as you rise, so take care.

4. To regress the stretch, come up onto your forearms rather than your hands.

5. To vary the stretch to work your obliques, simply lean to one side. Explore the positions to find the optimal stretch.

6. Hold for 30-60 seconds, or for 2 minutes if the musculature is very tense.

7. Complete 1-3 times.

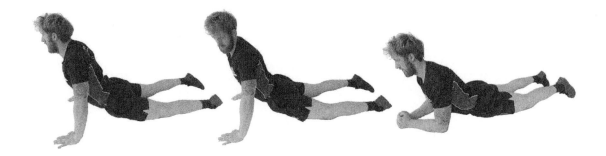

Hamstring Release Techniques & Stretches

If your hamstrings are excessively tight they can pull your pelvis into a posterior tilt, which in turn can flatten your back and cause back pain. If this is the case, hamstring stretches will be beneficial.

It's important to understand that your hamstrings may be tense because your pelvis has an anterior tilt which is pulling your hamstrings upwards. This is an example of when a muscle is in a lengthened state and tense.

If this is the case, stretching is not the best solution. Instead strengthening your hamstrings is the best approach (along with glutes and abs), while stretching the muscles that pull your pelvis into an anterior tilt, such as your hip flexors.

The hamstrings are also a good example of a muscle being chronically tight, not because of an issue with the hamstrings, but because there is a lack of core stability, or because your glutes aren't pulling their weight (hamstrings tighten to compensate). This goes to show that stretching a muscle that is tight, is not always the solution on its own, but can be an effective part of a complete solution.

The Biceps Femoris – One of the Hamstrings

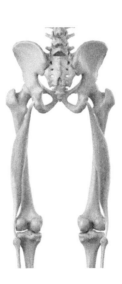

Hamstring Release Technique – Foam Rolling:

1. Sit on the floor and place a foam roller under the top of your right or left hamstring.

2. Both sides can be done at the same time if the roller is long enough. However, doing one at a time allows for more pressure to be placed through the hamstrings.

3. If rolling your right leg, place your left foot over your right and raise yourself up with your hands.

4. Slowly roll up and down the muscle for 30-60 seconds. Ensure you don't roll over the back of the knee, as there are structures in your knee crease (lymph nodes) that you don't want to drive a roller into. Focus on the bulk of the muscle.

5. Complete 1-2 times on each side.

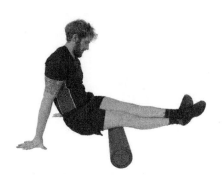

Hamstring Release Technique – Massage Ball:

A massage ball can be used to roll throughout the entire length of the hamstrings. However, this drill is designed specifically to reach the top of your hamstrings.

This can be specifically beneficial for those who have an anterior pelvic tilt, which pulls the hamstrings upwards causing excessive tension in the upper hamstrings.

1. Place the massage ball on a solid chair or platform.

2. Sit on the ball so that it is driven into the top of your hamstrings.

3. Knead the soft tissue and find any areas of excessive tension.

4. Apply pressure to an area of tension and slowly straighten and bend the knee.

5. Complete 1-2 sets of 5-10 reps on each leg.

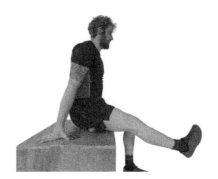

Standing Bilateral Stretch:

During any standing hamstring stretch it's important to understand that rounding your spine and dropping down to touch your toes isn't necessarily a true test of hamstring flexibility. You might have a mobile lower spine that allows you to bend over double.

1. Stand with your feet shoulder-width or slightly wider apart.

2. Keep your knees straight throughout. However, they don't have to be locked out, you can maintain a soft knee position.

3. Hinge at your hips by driving your glutes back, ensuring your knees don't bend and your chest remains proud.

4. As your glutes move back, you will feel the stretch on your hamstrings.

5. Hold for 30-60 seconds, or for 2 minutes if the musculature is very tense.

6. Complete 1-3 times.

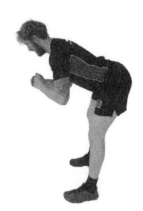

Seated Unilateral Stretch:

Here's an excellent stretch that can be done while sat at your desk.

1. Sit at the front of your chair.

2. Place your right leg straight out onto your heel.

3. Shift your glutes back slightly, tilting your pelvis forward. Do this correctly and you will feel the stretch in your hamstring.

4. Lean forward with your torso, ensuring you don't round your back.

5. Hold for 30-60 seconds, or for 2 minutes if the musculature is very tense.

6. Complete 1-3 times on each side.

A similar stretch can be done while standing, pictured below.

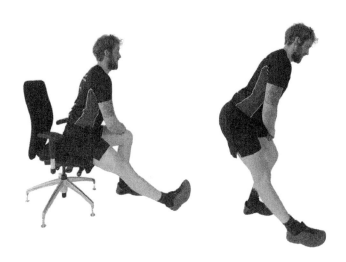

Lying Band Stretch:

Bands can be used effectively during many stretches.

1. Sit on the floor.

2. Place the resistance band around the arch of one foot, holding it with both hands.

3. Lie back so your head is flat to the floor. Maintain a neutral spine position.

4. Pull on the band to raise the leg up to facilitate the stretch.

5. Hold for 30-60 seconds, or for 2 minutes if the musculature is very tense.

6. Complete 1-3 times on each side.

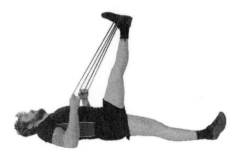

Adductor Release Technique & Stretches

The adductors are a large group of muscles on your inner thigh which are responsible for bringing your legs back toward your body from the side.

They oppose your hip abductors (gluteal muscles), and it's important that these groups are balanced. If the adductors are tight, it can inhibit your glutes and create back pain.

The adductors often get completely forgotten when training, simply because many women don't want to develop their inner thighs and most men generally pay more attention to their quads, calves, and hamstrings.

The Adductor Magnus – one of the adductors

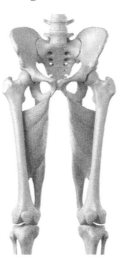

Adductor Release Technique – Foam Rolling:

When rolling, it's important to ensure that you try to cover the full length of the muscle. Often muscles will cross joints and areas which might not react well to having pressure placed on them. This can be due to the presence of things like neurovascular bundles - combinations of nerves, arteries, veins, and lymphatic vessels that travel together in the body.

Your groin is one area where caution must be practised. However, you can still roll throughout the length of the adductors effectively.

1. Lie face down on the floor with the roller to your side at your hips.

2. Raise the leg you are rolling out to the side and place your inner thigh on the roller.

3. If you can't raise your leg to the roller, simply lower it down, ensuring the roller ends up perpendicular to your leg.

4. Use your forearms to raise your body up to apply more pressure onto the foam roller.

5. Slowly roll up and down the muscle mass for 30-60 seconds.

6. Complete 1-2 times on each side.

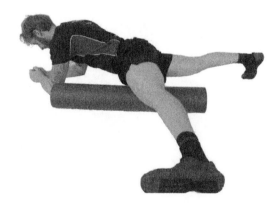

Extra Drill – Barbell Release Technique:

Foam rolling often requires you to hold yourself in taxing positions as you roll the targeted muscle(s). However, the weight of a barbell can be used to effectively roll muscles targeted while sitting.

This is an awesome technique to target your adductors and inner quad muscles.

1. Sit on the floor and place your left leg out to the side.

2. Place the sleeve of the barbell onto your inner thigh.

3. Slowly roll up and down the muscle mass for 30-60 seconds.

4. Complete 1-2 times on each side.

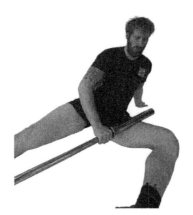

Seated Butterfly Stretch:

This is a simple but effective stretch for your adductors.

1. Sit on the floor and place the soles of your feet together.

2. Pull your heels in towards your groin.

3. Hold onto the balls of your feet.

4. Lean forward with your torso, keeping your spine straight, and push your knees towards the ground.

5. Hold for 30-60 seconds, or for 2 minutes if the musculature is very tense.

6. Complete 1-3 times on each side.

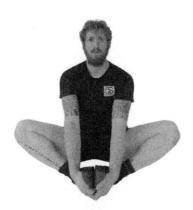

Deep Squat Stretch:

This is my favourite stretch for your lower body as it targets every muscle essential for achieving a deep squat.

I recommend spending as much time as you can in a deep squat, some experts prescribe at least 10 minutes a day.

1. Stand with your feet shoulder width apart. Toes can be angled out slightly (anywhere up to around 30 degrees).

2. Squat down into the deepest squat you can achieve. Try to maintain a neutral spine with a proud chest.

3. Some lumbar flexion (where your lower back rounds slightly as your pelvis tilts underneath) in a deep squat is normal, just ensure it is not excessive or putting stress on your lower back.

4. Place your hands into a prayer position and use your elbows to push your knees outwards.

5. Hold for 30-60 seconds, or for 2 minutes if the musculature is very tense.

6. Complete 1-3 times on each side.

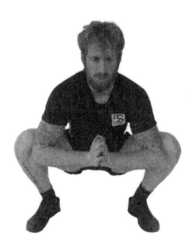

Chapter 6: Hip & Core Strength & Stability

Increasing hip and core strength is essential for maintaining the health of your entire body from head to toe.

Having weak hip and core muscles can cause countless issues, some of which can be life changing. Low back pain is a very common example of this.

I have worked with literally hundreds of clients who have suffered with what's commonly referred to as 'non-specific low back pain'. This is a general term that refers to any type of back pain in the lumbo-pelvic region that is not related to serious pathology and/or does not have a specific cause. Some disagree with the term, and I can understand why, as the diagnosis can often leave the sufferer with the feeling that there is no cause and therefore no remedy.

What has been proven time and time again to have the most benefits to this condition is strengthening and mobilising various muscles which surround and support the lumbar spine and pelvis. This, in turn, reinforces good posture, which should be consciously maintained as best possible throughout the day.

As with any injury, the onus is on you to maintain your own body. There are a number of injuries/ailments where certain exercises should not be used, and therefore specialist care is necessary. However, if you are suffering with low back pain after a long day sitting at your desk it's in your best interest to educate yourself as to how you can incorporate basic exercises to alleviate and rectify this discomfort.

Strength is essentially your ability to exert force, whereas stability is your ability to resist force. When we train, we often become very good at exerting force, but the muscles that help to resist force and stabilise movements can often get left behind.

The primary action of the core is to provide stability. You must first and foremost train your ability to resist the forces that are going to be applying stress to your spine.

There is some controversy around sit-up type exercises, which stems from the fact that repeated bending and twisting of the spine can result in the intervertebral disc fibres cracking and delamination occurring. However, there are many ways to effectively train the core without compromising the health of your lower spine.

While strength is essential for both good function and overall health of your structure, it's not effective to develop the muscles that stabilise your structure throughout the day as you would the muscles that facilitate large/explosive movements.

Large primary movers (lats, quads, pecs) respond well to high loads, which ultimately stimulates the greatest strength increases. However, the muscles which help to maintain stability require good endurance and respond well to isometric holds (where there is no change in muscle length i.e. a plank) or high reps with moderate weight. Overloading these muscles with weight can result in primary movers taking over.

Below is a series of strength and conditioning exercises that I use daily in my gym to help individuals achieve better posture, and better overall physical health and performance. Remember, performance refers to everything from elite level sport, to being able to carry out daily activities pain free.

Banded Glute Bridges, Frog Pumps & Lateral Band Walks

The glutes are made up of three major muscles, the gluteus maximus, medius, and minimus.

The gluteus maximus, or 'glute max', is the largest of the three and primarily works to extend your hips, making it incredibly important for standing up, running, and jumping.

The gluteus medius and minimus are the two smaller glutes which, along with the glute max, make up your buttocks. These two muscles facilitate various hip actions but also act to stabilise the hips and pelvis when the opposite leg is raised from the ground. It's clear to see why they are extremely important for low back and lower limb health.

It's common for the glutes to become underactive. When this is the case, we often prescribe glute activation exercises to get them working again.

It's important that we don't make the mistake of thinking everyone's glutes are inhibited and that glute activation is the key to all ailments involving the hips. However, most people can benefit from extra glute work, especially if the surrounding muscles are balanced.

You will notice below that the rep ranges are quite high. Ingraining a movement by repeating it many times is a great way to get a muscle 'firing' (a term commonly used to describe if a muscle is contracting how it should).

The Gluteus Maximus

The Gluteus Medius

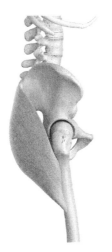
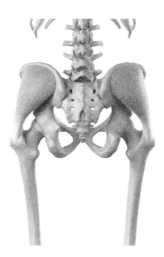

Banded Glute Bridges:

These can be performed without a band, but placing a band around your knees and abducting your legs (driving your knees apart), really helps to maximise the glute engagement as you extend your hips up from the floor.

1. Sit on the floor and place a small band around your legs, just above your knees.

2. Lie back so your head is flat to the floor.

3. Place your hands to the side.

4. Bend your knees and bring your heels towards your glutes. This prevents your hamstrings from taking over the work.

5. Place your feet flat to the floor, either together or hip width apart.

6. Spread your knees apart to abduct and externally rotate your hips.

7. Squeeze your glutes and extend your hips.

8. Hold at the top for 2-3 seconds before returning to the starting position.

9. Complete 3-5 sets of 20-30 reps.

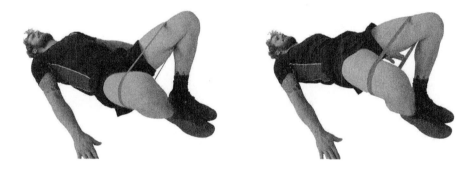

Above is the standard glute bridge set up. However, there are a few slight changes that can be made to help increase glute engagement.

Give them a go and see what works for you.

1. Tilt your pelvis by bringing your lower back flat to the floor.

2. Flex your head slightly, bringing your chin to your chest, rather than keeping it flat to the floor.

3. Coming up onto your heels and taking your toes off the floor.

4. Rather than having your palms flat to the floor, bend your elbows, clench your fists, and drive your arms into the floor.

Frog Pumps:

Frog pumps are a simple variation of the glute bridge.

1. Sit on the floor and lie onto your back.

2. Bend your knees. Keeping your heels close to your glutes to reduce hamstring engagement.

3. Incorporate the points mentioned previously that help to increase glute engagement.

4. Place the soles of your feet together and as close to your glutes as possible.

5. Squeeze your glutes and extend your hips.

6. A 1 second pause can be added at the top. However, frog pumps are usually carried out quickly.

7. Complete 3-5 sets of 20-50 reps.

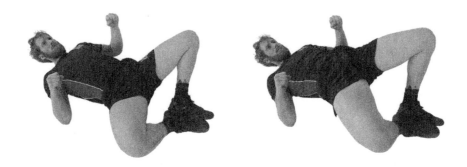

Lateral Band Walks:

Lateral band walks are a superb exercise for your glute medius, which is responsible for stabilising you while on one leg.

This drill can be done with a short band placed just above or below your knees, or with a long band using either the X-drill, or looping the whole band under the arches of your feet (my personal favourite).

1. Take a long band and hold it at either end in each hand.

2. Loop the band under the arches of your feet.

3. Stand up tall with good posture, bend your knees slightly.

4. Step 1-2 foot lengths to the right. Stay in control and don't allow your leg to be dragged by the band.

5. Complete 3-5 sets of 10-20 strides in each direction.

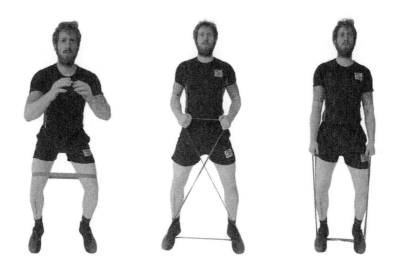

Banded Psoas March

The glutes are a hot topic when it comes to the need for activation and strengthening. Whereas the hip flexors are on the other end of the scale, with the need for mobility being the common prescription.

Prolonged sitting is often a huge factor in this. Sitting will weaken your glutes through underuse, while your hip flexors are kept in a flexed position, often causing them to tighten and become tense.

It's easy to see how keeping your hip flexors in a shortened position for extended periods can cause issues. However, an area that often becomes underworked is the full range of hip flexion, taking your hip past the 90-degree angle that a seated position usually keeps you in.

Therefore, while working your hip flexors, it's important to work them through full hip flexion and extension, to work the full range of motion and promote proper function. Remember, a weak muscle will often become a tense muscle.

1. Sit on the floor and place the band around the centre of your feet.

2. Lie back so your head is flat on the floor.

3. Bend your knees and raise your feet up, bringing your legs right back towards your torso.

4. Slowly extend your left leg, while ensuring your right leg remains in a fully flexed position.

5. Slowly return your left leg back to a flexed position and proceed to extend your right leg.

6. Complete 3-5 sets of 10-20 reps (counting each leg extension as a rep).

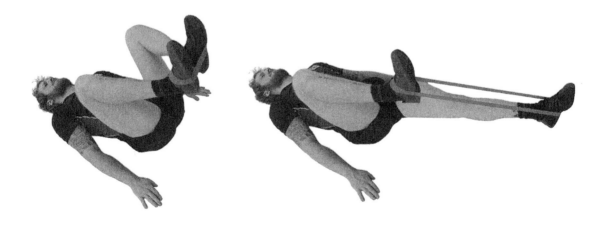

Dead Bug

The dead bug exercise is perfect for developing good posture as it requires you to work to maintain a neutral pelvis position while working your abs.

A key component of the dead bug exercise (along with the birddog exercise below), is that it incorporates both hip and shoulder function.

Individuals may have good hip function, however as soon as their shoulders come into play, it can throw their pelvis out of good posture. An example of this can be seen when someone with tight lats reaches overhead. As their lats don't allow a good overhead position, they often compensate by hyperextending their lower spine.

1. Lie on your back with your head flat on the floor.

2. Tilt your pelvis to flatten your lower back to the floor. Ensure you maintain this position throughout the exercise.

3. Extend your arms up to the front, with your palms facing forward.

4. Raise your feet up, bending your knees and hips at 90 degrees (this is your starting position).

5. Slowly extend your right leg to a point where your heel is just off the floor.

6. At the same time, flex your left arm to take it overhead, bringing it to a point where your hand is just off the floor.

7. Slowly return your leg and arm back to the starting position and proceed with the opposite sides.

8. Complete 3-5 sets of 10-20 reps (counting each leg extension as a rep).

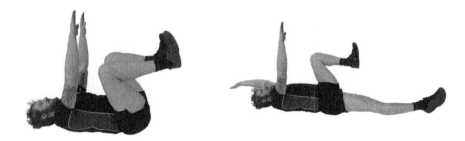

Birddog

The birddog exercise has a similar concept to the dead bug. However, you are working from all fours.

It's a great exercise for working your abs and back, again working both hip and shoulder function.

1. Start on all fours, with your elbows and shoulders over your hands and your hips over your knees.

2. Ensure your spine and pelvis stay neutral. Avoid tipping to one side to compensate.

3. Keep your core tight and slowly extend your right leg behind you while reaching forward with your left arm to the front (flexing your shoulder). This position can be held like a plank.

4. Return your arm and leg back to the starting position and proceed with the opposite side, or you can bring your left elbow (or palm) to your right knee before extending them out again without placing them down.

5. Complete 3-5 sets of 10-20 reps (counting each leg extension as a rep).

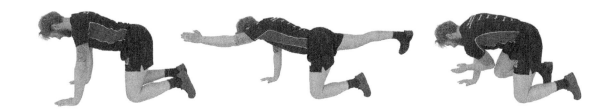

McGill Curl Up

McGill curls ups are named after Dr Stuart McGill who is a leading spinal researcher who promotes the use of what he refers to as 'the Big 3': McGill curl ups, birddogs, and side planks are his non-negotiable core exercises for a healthy lower spine.

McGill curl ups are essentially a sit up variation, which have the benefit of working your abs without excessively flexing your lumbar vertebra.

The exercise can look easy, but as with all core work, when it is performed correctly and you consciously engage the muscles you are trying to work, they are one of the hardest ab exercises out there.

1. Lie down with your head flat on the floor.

2. Bend your right leg, bringing your heel up towards your glutes while keeping your left leg extended.

3. Bend your elbows and place your hands under your lower back. This ensures you maintain a neutral spine throughout the movement. Keeping your elbows raised off the floor throughout the movement makes it harder.

4. Slowly raise your head and shoulders up a few inches and maximally contract your abs for 10 seconds before slowly returning to the starting position.

5. Try not to roll your chin towards your chest. Keep your chin retracted as you raise your shoulders and head up.

6. Complete 3-5 sets of 5 reps with 10 second pauses at the top.

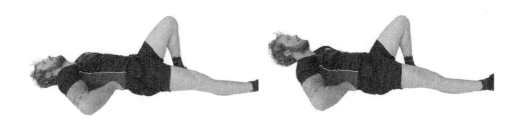

Ab Roll-Outs

Ab roll-outs work your abs incredibly hard while requiring you to maintain posture of your lumbo-pelvis region, making them one of the best core exercises in your arsenal.

The need to maintain a neutral pelvis and lower spine position while bending and extending your hips and knees makes the ab roll-out not only a great exercise for your abs, but also the ideal core exercise to ingrain proper function while squatting.

Caution must be practised with the ab roll-out as form can be easily lost, causing the lower back to dip and in some cases causing strains in the abs.

Many of your adductors connect to your pubis on your pelvis, which is the same area that your abdominals attach. Therefore, combining the engagement of these muscles with the ab roll-out will really work this complex of muscles that have a direct relationship with your pelvis, increasing the benefits.

To increase adductor engagement during the roll-out, simply place a medicine ball between your legs and squeeze your legs together as you roll out.

You can use an ab roller or even plates on a barbell.

1. Kneel with your hips stacked over your knees and grasp the roller/barbell.

2. Take a big gulp of air, while engaging your core musculature.

3. Slowly roll the roller out to the front and allow your body to extend. Ensure your lower spine doesn't dip.

4. Once your hips are fully extended or you have reached the furthest point your core strength allows, slowly return to the starting position.

5. Exhale.

6. Complete 3-5 sets of 5-10 reps (pauses can be used at the bottom).

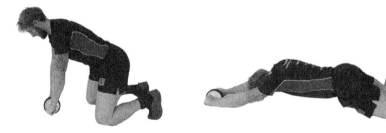

RKC Plank

Plank variations are isometric holds where your core musculature works to resist gravity as it pushes you into hyperextension and lateral flexion (side bending) of your spine.

The key to isometric core exercises is to consciously engage the musculature of the core, specifically your transverse abdominis (TVA).

The TVA is the deepest muscle of the abdominal wall and is an integral component of the core. It is often seen as the body's natural weight lifting belt, commonly being trained with the vacuum exercise.

The vacuum exercise involves drawing your belly button inward toward your spine. However, rather than performing this alone, we simply use the same technique while performing various exercises to engage the TVA.

The Transverse Abdominis

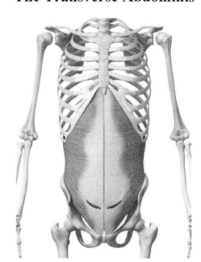

The RKC plank is named after the Russian Kettlebell Challenge by Pavel Tsatsouline, a famous Russian strength coach. It uses a few slight variations from the standard front plank while concentrating on engaging total body tension.

The RKC plank has been shown to get four times the ab engagement compared to the conventional front plank, and is my plank variation of choice.

You don't need to hold the RKC for minutes at a time. If you contract your core maximally, short rounds with even shorter rest periods work perfectly.

Often coaches will state that "if you can plank for a minute with ease, then you need to progress the exercise". I am sure this is true for planks where there is little to no conscious engagement, but if you maximally engage the associated musculature even 20-30 seconds will be enough for most.

1. Kneel on the floor, clasp your hands together so that your forearms are at a 45-degree angle.

2. Place your forearms onto the floor just as you would during a standard front plank. To increase the intensity, place your arms further forward so that your elbows sit in front of your shoulders.

3. Step back with your left then right foot at hip to shoulder width.

4. Maximally contract your glutes, which will tilt your pelvis back slightly.

5. Maximally contract your quads and core musculature. Pull back with your forearms to increase your core engagement.

6. Complete 3-5 sets of 30-40 seconds.

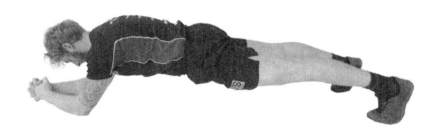

Side Planks

Side planks are a greatly underused exercise which are ideal for the development and maintenance of the deep core musculature that supports your spine and resists lateral flexion (side bending of the spine).

1. Sit on the floor.

2. Lie to the side and place your right forearm onto the floor, perpendicular to your body.

3. Placing your left foot to the front of your right foot, helps to keep your hips in a balanced position and also allows you to easily transition from front and side plank variations.

4. Raise your hips up so there is no side bending of your spine and your lower legs are raised off the floor.

5. Engage your glutes so your hips are extended. Having slightly bent hips is a common fault.

6. Maximally brace your core musculature as you would during a RKC plank.

7. Either keep your left arm flat to your body or raise it to the sky.

8. Complete 2-3 sets of 30-40 seconds on each side.

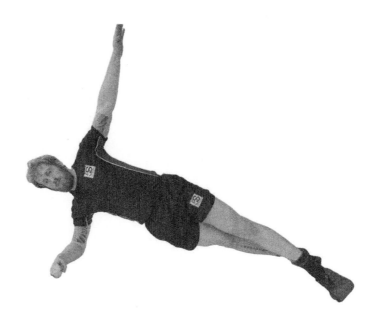

Pallof Iso Holds

This exercise is usually performed as a "pallof press" where you press the resistance band rather than sustaining an isometric hold. However, the pallof iso hold is my favourite anti-rotation exercise.

The pallof iso hold can be performed in various stances while standing or kneeling. These variations should be practised as it will help to build lumbo-pelvic stability in various positions.

1. Use a red band. The tension can be varied by standing closer to, or further away from the band attachment point if required.

2. Attach the band to something solid at chest height, looping the band through itself.

3. Grasp the band with both hands and stand side-on to the attachment point, holding your hands at your chest.

4. Side step away from the attachment point to add tension to the band.

5. Ensure that your feet, hips and shoulders are forward facing. Don't counter the band tension by turning away from the attachment point.

6. If performing the pallof press, engage your core and press the band to your front, holding it for 2-5 seconds before returning it to the starting position and proceeding with successive reps.

7. For an isometric hold, press the band out and hold it for 30-40 seconds.

8. Complete 2-3 sets of 5-15 reps or 30-40 seconds on each side.

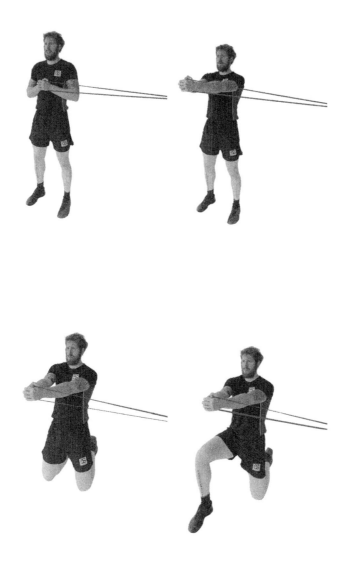

Hip Hinges

All the previous exercises are designed to target and work specific areas of the hips and core. The next three exercises also develop these areas, but the main emphasis is developing proper movement.

For example, the protocol for someone suffering with low back pain, may often be to increase core and glute strength to help reduce the load on their lower spine. However, it's also essential to retrain proper movement.

The hip hinge involves bending at your hips to allow your torso to drop forward while maintaining a neutral spine (unbent and untwisted). It is an essential movement pattern that will allow you to perform daily tasks, like picking an object up off the ground, without compromising your back.

The hinge is truly the foundation of good movement. People often think that you must perfectly squat down to correctly pick up an object, but this is completely unrealistic. There is nothing wrong with bending over (hinging at your hips) if the muscles that support the movement are working correctly and you maintain good posture throughout.

People often make the argument, "well a baby always squats down to pick something up". This is true, but babies have extremely short legs in relation to their long torso, and if you know anything about squat mechanics, that's the perfect ratios for deep squatting. Adults on the other hand tend to come in all shapes and sizes and some simply can't achieve a full depth squat.

Your hips, like your shoulders, are ball-and-socket joints and should facilitate many actions such as bending over to pick something up. Problems occur when these actions are repeatedly facilitated with bending movements of the spine.

I will first describe how to correctly perform a hip hinge before showing you one of the best barbell movements for hinge development.

Bodyweight Hinge:

1. Stand with soft knees and good upper body posture, ensuring your chest is proud and remains so throughout the movement.

2. Start by driving your glutes back. Standing a foot length from a wall and attempting to touch the wall with your glutes works as an ideal teaching aid.

3. Maintain the soft knee position and keep driving your glutes back, this will cause your hips to hinge, dropping your torso forward.

4. Keep going until you feel your hamstrings reach the extent of their range of motion. Ensure you maintain a neutral spine.

5. With straight legs (soft knees) and maintaining a neutral spine, this will usually bring your torso to parallel or just above parallel to the floor.

6. Complete 3-5 sets of 10 reps.

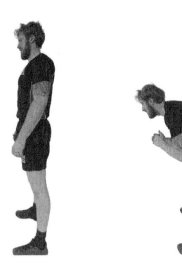

RDL – Romanian Deadlift:

The Romanian deadlift was developed by a Romanian weightlifter named Nicu Vlad.

He was seen by some American lifters in a gym in San Francisco doing a lift that looked like a cross between the stiff legged deadlift and the conventional deadlift (the most commonly used technique for picking a barbell up off the floor).

Someone watching asked what the lift was called and after he replied that he didn't have a name for it, they came up with the name Romanian deadlift or RDL for short – that story isn't integral to the exercise, but people always ask, "why Romanian?", and now you know.

It is a great lift that can be done with dumbbells. However, it is best done with a barbell as it allows for the most weight to be incrementally lifted.

The RDL is my lift of choice when progressing individuals from a bodyweight hinge to working with weight. It acts as a great prerequisite to the deadlift, which involves pulling the barbell up off the floor.

1. The starting position for this lift is with the barbell at your hips with a pronated grip (overhand), so ensure you pick the barbell up with good form, maintaining a neutral spine.

2. Initiate the movement by driving your glutes back and bending your knees slightly. Allow your shoulders to come over the barbell while the barbell maintains contact with your legs.

3. Keep driving your glutes back to facilitate the hinge and allow the barbell to track down your quads. If there is too much knee bend at this point, the barbell will sit on your quads, rather than tracking down smoothly.

4. Once the barbell passes your knee caps, bend your knees slightly to bring the barbell to about a palms distance below your knees.

5. Engage the glutes and bring the barbell back up your legs in the same path it came down. Maintain a vertical bar path throughout (if you were to watch someone from the side, you would see the barbell go up and down in a vertical line).

6. Squeeze your glutes hard at the top to really get them firing and proceed with successive reps.

7. Depending on the weight being used, complete 3-5 sets of 5-8 reps.

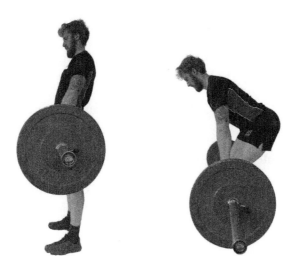

Squats

The ability to squat well is considered the epitome of functional movement and strength development. It is a fundamental movement, one that is utilised countless times a day.

You might not think you are required to squat, but every time you bend and straighten your knees and hips, you are working the muscles that the squat trains.

Squats are simply the most effective way of developing your leg strength, and ingraining the correct form and sequence to help keep you in good health while performing daily tasks.

The reason squats work so well is because they involve taking your hips, knees, and ankles into a decent degree of flexion before returning up into an extended position, while maintaining a neutral spine.

In this section, I will introduce the body weight squat and my personal favourite variation for teaching the movement - the goblet squat.

The capacity of the legs is huge, so it is beneficial to introduce weight to your training. A common phrase is 'the mind will give in before the legs'. This speaks truth, since the legs are built to hold the weight of your body and potentially carry it for miles each day.

There seems to be a lot of debate regarding the correct depth for a squat. Some believe it necessary to go 'ass to grass', where you drop to a depth where their knees are fully bent. Others however, favour a depth where their hamstrings are parallel or just below to the floor.

Things like joint anatomy and limb lengths can play a key role in the way people squat. However, the level of depth I consider ideal involves squatting just below parallel, where the crease of your hips just surpass the top of your knee caps.

This position maximises muscle engagement while placing the least maladaptive stress on the rest of your body, specifically your knees and lumbar spine.

Bodyweight Squat:

1. Take a shoulder width stance with your toes pointing slightly outwards (no more than 30 degrees).

2. Initiate the movement with your hips, driving your glutes back.

3. Bend your knees as your hips hinge (almost simultaneously).

4. Lower under control, pushing your knees outwards if they have a tendency of falling inwards (valgus). Your knees want to stay in line with your toes.

5. As you squat, bring your hands to your front. This acts as a counter balance as your centre of mass moves back.

6. Squat down to the appropriate depth (ideally breaking parallel).

7. At full depth (often referred to as 'the hole'), your knees will more-than-likely sit directly over your toes. Limb lengths can vary this, but you don't want your knees to move too far beyond your toes, as it places a lot of stress on them.

1. Capitalise on the stretch reflex (involuntary contraction in response to a stretch in the muscles) to help you recoil out of the hole (bottom of the squat), and drive back up out of the squat.

8. Complete 3-5 sets of 10-20 reps.

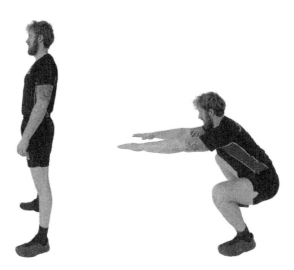

Goblet Squat:

As mentioned previously, the goblet squat is excellent for perfecting squat mechanics. This is because holding a weight to your front as you squat acts as a perfect counter balance.

The exercise was developed by strength coach Dan John and was named after the position in which the weight is held, up high at the chest as if you are holding a large goblet.

When novices perform bodyweight squats they often have little depth and excessive forward tilt of their torso, many coaches will jump in to try to rectify any mobility issues the individual may have. However, stability is often the underlying problem. If a muscle is tight, the first question is whether it's due to a lack of stability.

To test this, a coach should give the novice a weight to hold to the front, and the goblet position makes for a perfect counterbalance. This takes away many of the stability issues they may be suffering from and allows for decent depth to be achieved as their torso remains more upright.

It can literally progress someone with a terrible bodyweight squat, to squatting well within just one set.

A kettlebell is usually used, but a dumbbell or a weight plate also work well.

2. Squat down and grasp the handle of the kettlebell with both hands.

3. Lift the kettlebell and set up your stance just as you would for a bodyweight squat.

4. Keep your elbows in on either side of the kettlebell so that when you squat down, they comfortably fit in between your legs.

5. Perform the squat as you would a bodyweight squat, allowing the kettlebell to work as a counter balance.

6. Depending on the weight being used, complete 3-5 sets of 5-20 reps.

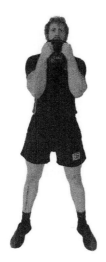
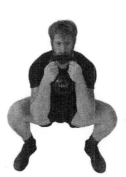

Lunges

Lunges are essentially a single leg squatting action and often you will hear people describe variations of these movements as both 'split squats' and 'lunges'.

The lunge and split squat are very similar at first glance, however there is a small difference.

During a lunge, both legs, regardless of their positioning, are involved in completing the movement. Usually the front 'plant' leg is holding around 75% of the weight, while the rear 'supporting' leg is holding around 25%.

During a split squat on the other hand, only one leg is utilised to complete the movement, while the other leg is pretty much at rest, applying a small degree of support.

Lunges can be performed forwards, backwards and laterally out to the side, either moving in one direction (walking lunge) or in an alternating fashion where you return to the same starting position each time.

Forwards/Rearwards Lunge:

A forward stride into a lunge is most often used simply because it is what comes naturally. However, a forward striding lunge does place quite a lot of stress on the front knee. Therefore, if you have knee pain or find the forward lunge stressful, I would recommend using a backwards stride, which helps to unload a lot of the stress.

There are a few foot placement variations that can be used during lunges. I suggest using a semi-inline stance, where the feet line up to the side of each other with little or no gap between them from a front view. It's fine to go wider than this if you require extra stability, however, an excessively straddled stance can apply stress to your groin.

The semi-inline stance provides a stable foot placement, while maintaining optimal mechanics for the hip joints and the musculature of the lower body.

Lunges can be loaded with a barbell. However, people usually use a dumbbell in each hand at their sides.

1. Start with a hip width foot placement.

2. Take a reasonably long stride with your right leg which allows your left knee to drop comfortably towards the floor while your right knee tracks forward slightly but is still behind your toes

3. It is fine for your left knee to gently touch the floor. However, this is often avoided to ensure tension remains throughout your body and you don't strike your knee causing bruising - I suggest taking your knee to 1 inch off the floor.

4. As you stride with the front leg and your knee bends, a slight hip hinge will ensure the movement maximises the engagement of not only your quads, but also your hamstrings and glutes. This also ensures your knee doesn't move too far forwards.

5. If completing an alternate lunge, stride back to the original starting position, but if you are doing a walking lunge, stride forward into the next lunge with the opposite leg.

6. During walking lunges, you can set the recovering leg down before striding out with it into the next lunge, or pass it straight past the supporting leg and into the next lunge.

7. Depending on the weight being used, complete 3-5 sets of 8-20 reps.

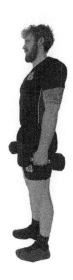 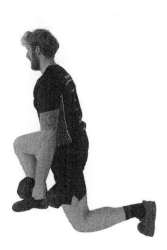

Lateral Lunge:

This is a lunge variation where you stride out to the side keeping the non-striding leg straight.

This variation both mobilises and strengthens your adductors, which are normally overlooked when it comes to training. However, as you know from the previous section on adductors, if ignored they can cause all sorts of problems that will need addressing.

The lateral lunge can be performed from a pre-set starting position where your legs are spread at the distance required to lunge with good form, or you can start from a hip-width stance and stride sideways into the wider stance before dropping into the lunge.

I will be describing the lunge performed from the pre-set stance.

A barbell can be used with this movement. However, I recommend using a kettlebell in a goblet position.

1. Take a wide stance that allows you to facilitate the lunge. This may need adjusting when you try the first rep.

2. Keep your toes forward facing and stay on the soles of your feet throughout the whole movement.

3. Bend your left knee and drive your glutes back to facilitate a hinge.

4. Full depth is achieved when you feel a full stretch on your adductors. Don't roll onto the side of your right foot.

5. Depending on the weight being used, complete 3-5 sets of 8-20 reps.

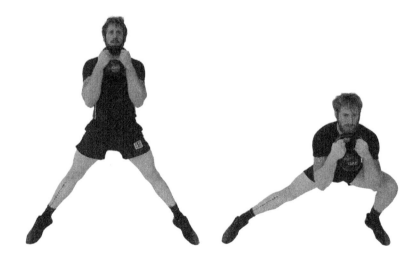

Chapter 7: Programming

Introduction

This chapter takes the information from the previous sections and brings it together to create effective programmes.

Some of these are mobility routines you can carry out at your desk, while others are whole workouts designed for at home or in the gym.

The exercises in this book can be put together in any way that suits your specific needs. However, some exercise combinations complement each other well, so start with the programmes I have created and develop from there.

Not every exercise in the book has been included, but you can add them in where necessary as you develop your own workouts.

You can incorporate applicable release techniques (such as foam rolling) prior to any stretches.

At Your Desk

The following exercises can be performed while sat at your desk. I will incorporate lower body mobility in the next section as some of those exercises will be best carried out with some floor space.

These routines are specifically designed as short drills which you can do throughout the day.

Upper Body Mobility Regime:

Exercise	Sets/Reps/Time	Rest	Notes
Neck Extensor Stretch	1x20 Seconds	5 Seconds	
Levator Scapula Stretch	1x20 Seconds – Each side	5 Seconds	
Trapezius Stretch	1x20 Seconds – Each side	5 Seconds	
Scalene and Sternocleidomastoid Stretch	1x20 Seconds – Each side	5 Seconds	
Seated Chest Stretch	1x30 Seconds	5 Seconds	
Seated Thoracic Rotations	1x30 Seconds – Each side	5 Seconds	

Workout:

Ideally you should complete this short workout every 40-60 minutes if sitting for prolonged periods.

Exercise	Sets/Reps/Time	Rest	Notes
Seated Shoulder Rolls	1x5 Rolls – Each side	5 Seconds	
Head Retractions	1x5 Reps	5 Seconds	
Scapula Pinches	1x5 Reps	5 Seconds	
Seated Thoracic Rotations	1x20 Seconds – Each side	5 Seconds	
Seated Shoulder Rolls	1x5 Rolls – Each side	5 Seconds	

At Home/Office

These programmes can be incorporated into your gym routine, but you don't need gym equipment to complete them.

Mobility Regime – Upper Body:

Exercise	Sets/Reps/Time	Rest	Notes
Trapezius Stretch	2x20 Seconds – Each side	5 Seconds – 30 Seconds between exercises	
Standing Chest Stretch - Door	2x30 Seconds – Each side	5-10 Seconds	
Kneeling Lat Stretch	2x30 Seconds	5-10 Seconds	
Thoracic Extension Drill on Foam Roller	2x30 Seconds	5-10 Seconds	
Quadruped Thoracic Rotations	2x5 Reps – Each side	5 Seconds	

Mobility Regime – Hips & Core:

Exercise	Sets/Reps/Time	Rest	Notes
Figure Four Glute Stretch	2x30 Seconds – Each side	5-10 Seconds – 30 Seconds between exercises	
Cobra Stretch	2x30 Seconds	5-10 Seconds	
Kneeling Hip Flexor Stretch	2x30 Seconds – Each side	5-10 Seconds	
Hip Rolls	1x10 – Each side	5-10 Seconds	
Iron Cross Stretch	1x10 Reps – Each side	5-10 Seconds	

Shoulder External Rotation & Retraction:

Exercise	Sets/Reps/Time	Rest	Notes
Large Band External Rotations	3x10 – Each side	10-15 Seconds – 60 Seconds between exercises	
Standard Band Pull Apart	3x10	15-20 Seconds	
Band Face Pulls	3x10	15-20 Seconds	
Serratus Wall Slides	3x10	20-30 Seconds	

Hip & Core Strength & Stability:

Exercise	Sets/Reps/Time	Rest	Notes
Banded Glute Bridges	3x20 Reps	15-20 Seconds – 60 Seconds between exercises	
Dead Bug	1x10 Reps – Each side	20-30 Seconds	
Ab Roll Outs	3x5 Reps	20-30 Seconds	
RKC Plank	3x30 Seconds	15-20 Seconds	
Side Planks	2x30 Seconds – Each Side	15-20 Seconds	

Whole Body Workout:

Exercise	Sets/Reps/Time	Rest	Notes
Dead Bug	1x10 Reps – Each side	20-30 Seconds – 60 Seconds between exercises	
Birddog	1x10 Reps – Each side	20-30 Seconds	
Bodyweight Hip Hinge	4x10 Reps	20-30 Seconds	
Bodyweight Squat	4x10 Reps	20-30 Seconds	
Bodyweight Lunge	4x5 Reps – Each side	20-30 Seconds	
Band Pull Apart	3x10 Reps	20-30 Seconds	

In the Gym

Upper Body:

Exercise	Sets/Reps/Time	Rest	Notes
Star Pattern Band Pull Apart	3x15 Reps	15-20 Seconds – 60 Seconds between exercises	
Band Face Pulls	3x10 Reps	20-30 Seconds	
Bent Over Rows	4x10 Reps	60-90 Seconds	
Single Arm Rows	4x10 Reps – Each side	60-90 Seconds	
Shrugs	4x10 Reps	60-90 Seconds	
Band Horizontal Pulls - Bilateral	3x20 Reps	60 Seconds	

Lower Body:

Exercise	Sets/Reps/Time	Rest	Notes
Banded Glute Bridges	3x20 Reps	15-20 Seconds – 60 Seconds between exercises	
Banded Psoas March	3x10 Reps – Each side	15-20 Seconds	
Goblet Squats	4x10 Reps	60-90 Seconds	
RDL's	4x6 Reps	60-90 Seconds	
Weighted Lunges	4x10 Reps	60-90 Seconds	
Lateral Lunges	4x5 Reps – Each side	60-90 Seconds	

Core:

Exercise	Sets/Reps/Time	Rest	Notes
Ab Roll Outs	3x5 Reps	20-30 Seconds – 60 Seconds between exercises	
McGill Curl Ups	3x5 Reps	20-30 Seconds	
RKC Plank	3x30 Seconds	15-20 Seconds	
Side Planks	2x30 Seconds – Each Side	15-20 Seconds	
Pallof Iso Holds	2x40 Seconds – Each side	15-20 Seconds	

Whole Body Workout:

Exercise	Sets/Reps/Time	Rest	Notes
Banded Glute Bridges	3x20 Reps	15-20 Seconds – 60 Seconds between exercises	
Goblet Squats	4x10 Reps	60-90 Seconds	
Lateral Lunges	4x5 Reps – Each side	60-90 Seconds	
Standard Band Pull Apart	3x10 Reps	15-20 Seconds	
Bent Over Rows	4x10 Reps	60-90 Seconds	
Single Arm Rows	4x10 Reps – Each Side	60-90 Seconds	
Ab Roll Outs	3x5 Reps	20-30 Seconds	
RKC Plank	3x30 Seconds	15-20 Seconds	

Be Social!

Get in touch if you have any questions:

Facebook: 5sfitnessuk

Instagram: 5s_fitness